SHIPS *of* MERCY

THE REMARKABLE FLEET BRINGING HOPE
TO THE WORLD'S FORGOTTEN POOR

Don Stephens
with
Lynda R. Stephenson

Hodder & Stoughton
LONDON SYDNEY AUCKLAND

First published in Great Britain in 2005

10 9 8 7 6 5 4 3 2 1

British Library Cataloguing in Publication Data
A record for this book is available from the British Library

ISBN 0 340 86336 6

Printed and bound in Great Britain by
Bookmarque Ltd, Croydon, Surrey

The paper and board used in this paperback are natural recyclable products made
from wood grown in sustainable forests. The manufacturing processes conform
to the environmental regulations of the country of origin.

Hodder & Stoughton
A Division of Hodder Headline Ltd
338 Euston Road
London NW1 3BH
www.madaboutbooks.com
www.hodderbibles.co.uk

This book is dedicated to each who has been a part of our history, who has served so willingly, offering so much to those who have so little.

THANK YOU.

CONTENTS

CONTENTS

FOREWORD

Many years ago, Don and Deyon Stephens had a dream. They wished to help those who were unimaginably poor, living in meagre surroundings with no medical care and little hope for the future.

The modern world had passed these people by: no doctors, no dentists, no hospitals, no drugs, no alleviation of pain and no treatment of ailments. The reality of this bleak life inspired Don and Deyon to one of the most remarkable charities I know: Mercy Ships.

The Mercy Ships are hospital ships. They sail into the poorest parts of the world and they dock. They then set about curing men, women and children who expected to bear pain and discomfort all the days of their lives. In essence, Mercy Ships brings hope to those who had none.

I was introduced to Mercy Ships some years ago by my friend, and eminent surgeon, Ian McColl. I was captured immediately by the enthusiasm of the Mercy Ships volunteers and was honoured to become their Patron.

Each and every one of those who serve on board – from the surgeons and medical staff to the cooks and telephone operators – are volunteers. Most of the surgical staff, who lead hectic and stressful lives in their home countries, devote what little holiday periods they have to the work of these extraordinary floating hospitals.

Mercy Ships is based on the Christian ethic of service to the needy. Because of Mercy Ships, people see – who would be blind; walk – who would be crippled; live – who would die.

The dream that Don and Deyon once had is now a reality, and this book sets out the story of how it all came about. It is an inspiring tale of courage, fortitude and achievement, and no one who reads it could fail to be moved.

JOHN MAJOR, British Prime Minister 1990–1997
December 2004

SHIP OF HOPE

by Lord Ian McColl, MD, excerpted from *Reader's Digest*, UK, April 2002

 Dateline: Banjul, The Gambia
13°28′ N 16°40′ W

'*I need a Jolls retractor*,' *I said, expecting it to be slapped into my hand.*
'*We don't have one!*' *said the nurse.*
'*Well, what have you got?*'
'*I can give you a pair of hands.*'

So began our first stint with the international charity Mercy Ships ...
For the next two weeks, we stopped operating only to eat and (briefly) to sleep. I'm professor of surgery at Guy's Hospital in London, but I hadn't operated so intensively and for so long since I was a young houseman [intern], and I loved it. To slow down was unthinkable ... Daily, people streamed up the gangway for plastic surgery and eye treatments – infants born with cleft palate, faces bulging with tumours, children grossly disfigured ... people of all ages blinded by cataracts. For many, the Mercy Ship was their only hope ...

According to a hawker outside the Gambian wharf gates, local people came every night to gaze at the white ship bathed in her halo of light: 'They say they can see angels on her decks.'

Usually it's easy to feel overwhelmed by the needs of the Third World – with roughly one in four of the world's population having no access to formal medical care. But what we saw onboard the Anastasis transformed our notions of what ordinary people can do. From captains, surgeons and accountants to lab technicians, cooks and engine-room greasers, every person is not only a volunteer working round the clock, but is paying to do it . . .

With everyone doing their bit, and a bit more, heroic operations that would cost thousands of pounds in Europe can be done for next to nothing. Well over 5,000 people had lined up in the sweltering sun in a football stadium for screening day. During the ship's stay, nearly 800 patients had come down her gangway dancing on sunshine. This was a ship that carried that rare, most valuable commodity: a cargo of mercy . . .

SHIP'S LOG: JANUARY 2005

Newcastle, England
55°2' N 1°42' W

INTRODUCTION
A TALE TO TELL

A ship with 'a cargo of mercy – '

Patients coming down her gangway 'dancing on sunshine – '

Those great images expressed by Lord McColl, one of the UK's foremost surgeons, come to mind as I stand aloft on 'monkey island', fifty feet above the deck of the 20th century's newest Mercy Ship, the *Africa Mercy*. Below me is the world's largest nongovernmental hospital ship sailing the modern world's seas – six operating theatres, a seventy-eight-bed recovery ward, a women's ward, a limb-fitting centre, and living space for more than 484 volunteers and crew.

This newest cargo of mercy is almost on its way, and we can hardly wait to have more 'sunshine-dancing' down our gangways.

The nautical signal flags are up.

The captain is on the state-of-the-art command bridge.

All is ready for the latest Mercy Ship to set sail.

The view from up here is breathtaking. The sea air fills my senses and the snap of the flags above me is exhilarating. But it's not the sea air that is giving me chills: This moment has been more than twenty-five years in the making. And I am in awe of how I came to be standing right here – how millions have been touched through our ships' efforts, how thousands have danced down gangways into new lives, and thousands more of us have been privileged to make it so.

Imagine a fleet of hospital ships, staffed with professionals at the highest level of expertise from every nation – including doctors, dentists, nurses, teachers, cooks, seamen, and engineers – volunteering to sail to the planet's neediest ports to serve the forgotten poor, offering all their expertise without regard to race, colour, sex, or creed. That was what I'd imagined so long ago.

Most such ideas fade away with time. This one didn't. And I found myself day after day, year after year, in the middle of an idea that would not let me go. Until one day my imagined crew came to life before my eyes and, amazingly, made the dream set sail.

Some came for a career, some for two-year hitches, and many for shorter volunteer stretches of service to change the world by putting love into action in small ways or big ways. And they continue to come, filling ship waiting lists; shaping the future as they wait.

Twenty-five years ago, all we had was a dream. But it was a powerful dream. And it is a dream that continues, every day, to come true.

We have sailed to the edges of the poorest continents, bringing hope and healing; working in the same spirit that guided Mother Teresa and founded the Salvation Army and the Red Cross.

And in these places, the hospital ships have become part legend. That, I could never have imagined. But three generations now talk about the day the Mercy Ship came into port to give a transforming surgery on the child now a parent or the adult now a grandparent. The stories were told and told and told. And as the word spread over the years, medical screening days in the selected developing world ports became so large that governments began to open stadiums to hold the crowds. And as the legend grows, we grow to live up to it.

The numbers alone can take my breath away – more than 2 million services valued at more than 250 million dollars, with more than 5.5 million people in ninety-five ports in fifty-three developing nations. On land, more than 300,000 people have been treated in village medical and dental clinics, and over 5,500 local workers trained to instruct thousands of others in primary health care.

I could also quote you numbers about the need, numbers such as 1 billion people living in absolute poverty, their total energies every single day consumed with just staying alive. But such numbers are staggering to the point of our being unable to hear them, much less comprehend them. And the numbers don't say what we need and want to hear: What can we do? How can we help? What is possible to do in an increasingly impossible world?

It was easy to be overwhelmed twenty-five years ago; it still is today because even after helping so many, there are so many more. And we realise that even with this new, mighty 21st-century ship we'll never reach more than a tiny portion of those in need.

So why bother at all? Why do we continue to set sail?

Standing here, feeling not only the hum of the mechanical energy that runs the ship but also feeling the wonderful human energy as well, I can think of several good answers. But maybe the best answer comes from one of Lord McColl's tiniest patients, a little girl who told her new Mercy Ship friends how she liked to rescue starfish stranded on the beach and put them back in the ocean. When someone pointed out the futility of such action in the grand scheme of things, she said: 'It makes a difference to the starfish.'

Every man, woman, and child who find themselves, by accident of birth and culture and geography, out of reach of even the very basics of modern medicine, are like those starfish. We know this deep in our own souls: Every life is worthy. The best inside us wants to offer the best to others. Behind every statistic, there's a person in need of hope and healing. Every one's a story. Some heart wrenching, some heart stirring – none, though, you can ever forget.

Their stories and our story – the twenty-five-year saga of how an improbable idea launched Mercy Ships and continues to keep her afloat – are the same story. And it is the one I want to share.

The saga of Mercy Ships is the sometimes astonishing, sometimes crazy, sometimes outright providential history of the last quarter of a century. It's filled with intrigue and mistakes, world leaders and earthly saints, the drama of life and death, the stories of horrors of war and the resilience of the human spirit; and the miracles of modern medicine, human kindness and ingenuity.

In other words, it's a tale to tell.

Full steam ahead –

THE STORY OF EDOH

Dateline: Lome, Togo
6°10' N 1°21' E

She's tall and slender, sixteen going on seventeen, a French-speaking African young woman with the blood of three nations in her veins, or so it was eight years ago, when a younger Edoh underwent several surgical procedures and blood transfusions from crew members onboard a Mercy Ship.

She was nine at the time, a tiny child with spindly arms and legs and a massive tumour on the side of her face. The renegade mass had shifted her left eye two inches off centre and stretched her mouth to an unimaginable eight-inch diametre. Teeth stuck out at odd angles, and worse, a new backward growth of the tumour threatened a slow and horrible death by suffocation.

In shock and horror, her parents, having exhausted every possible avenue of hope, finally gave up. They, along with their village, prepared for her death. And then her parents heard that a Mercy Ship was coming.

Edoh remembers only the blood she would cough up, the difficulty breathing, the fear in her parents' eyes. She remembers too, the day they travelled a long way to stand in line, how she suddenly began fighting for breath, how she was snatched up from the press of a huge crowd and tossed screaming over a steel gate. She remembers landing in the arms of a giant white man and screaming more until she finally saw her parents again, inside the big ship on the other side of the fence.

Years have now passed, and the Mercy Ship has docked once again in Togo. Edoh has returned for a follow-up small reconstructive surgery, and everything comes flooding back to her, especially the care and the kindness of the nurses and the surgeons. She understood nothing of their speech, then, or now. But there is no forgetting the language of their touch.

And when she does find someone to translate her words, she tells them all she wants to become a nurse.

SHIP'S LOG: 1964–1977

Olathe, Colorado
38°36' N 107°58' W

Nassau, Bahamas
25°5' N 77°21' W

Lausanne, Switzerland
46°32' N 6°39' E

CHAPTER 1

THE BIRTH OF A DREAM

The most pathetic person in the world is someone who has sight but has no vision. – HELEN KELLER

I could say it all started with a hurricane, or reading a book about the famous SS *Hope*. I could say it started with meeting Mother Teresa, or with the birth of our special-needs son, John Paul. Or I could say it began with my parents' simple way with grace and mercy and dignity with their small-town helping hand. I could say all those things about the very beginning of the idea that became Mercy Ships, and they'd all be true.

Certain ideas and opportunities fall into place in providential ways in almost every life. As I look back at my own, I can see the patterns of things happening when they did, and why, and I find myself shaking my head at the wonder, the sheer improbability, of it all.

I had been imagining the idea of a hospital ship since I was nineteen, and considering I grew up in landlocked Colorado, that was rather odd, to say the least. Growing up in the fifties and sixties, I was part of a generation who wanted to change the world and believed it was possible. President Kennedy's Peace Corps was a popular and inspiring organisation. By the time I left home, I was already primed to think in terms of spending a life in some sort of humanitarian effort, just through watching my no-nonsense parents. My mother and father were the perfect blend for the western Colorado farming and ranching town of Olathe where I grew up.

With my mother, it was care and compassion; with my father,

practicality and integrity. My mother believed the best of everyone, and my father could spot a phoney a hundred yards away. My mother had a remarkable heart for helping needy families in our town, and a talent for treating them with dignity and respect that I quickly noticed as a child. 'You never know when I might be in that situation and you can help me,' was one of the phrases she used to put everyone at ease.

My father, on the other hand, a farmer, rancher, and a grocery-store owner was a pure, plain-spoken western man. What you saw was what you got. You never had to worry about what my dad thought, because he would tell you. And he told us a lot. 'Words come too easily for some people,' he'd say. 'I am far more interested in what you do, the deeds of your life, than any words you will ever say.'

That came home to me in a big way at his funeral. After the service, one of my parents' longtime friends asked if I knew why so many Mexican Americans were there. Many of those attending the memorial service were Hispanic, some people I'd never met.

'They were migrant workers,' my mother said. 'They tried to stay through the entire year, after harvest, and their families were close to starvation. Your father extended them credit when no other store owner would.' What was not being said was the obvious fact that they were people of integrity who paid him back, and, something better, they had passed on the story of his actions through their family life, honouring his good deed by making it part of their family lore. When you offer something life-affirming to someone who has nothing, the purest way they can honour the deed is to pass the story from one generation to the next. That fact echoed through my heart and soul years later when I heard how Mercy Ship stories became family legends, too.

So in 1964, at nineteen, I was raring to change the world, like so many others in my generation. I tagged along on a trip to the

Caribbean, organised by a group that has been described as a faith-based Peace Corps – an organisation called Youth With A Mission that corralled a lot of us teenagers to be part of a programme called SOS, a Summer of Service. What we didn't know was that we were walking right into a hurricane.

Back then there was no way to know when a hurricane was brewing – no warning, and no way to call anyone. All phone lines were down. Before I knew it, I was huddled with others in an aircraft hangar, riding out the worst of Hurricane Cleo as it roared around us. In the streets of Nassau, palm trees were being blown down, roofs blown off, and streets flooded. We were gathered in different venues for safety.

I was with a group in an old British World War II aircraft hangar that had withstood several storms. I remember cracking open those big hanger doors and staring at the sight. As you might imagine, we were all praying and praying hard. We were worried about ourselves and about our worried parents, and as the wind rattled and shook that hangar until it almost blew away itself, we couldn't help but think about the Bahamians losing their houses and livelihoods and some their very lives. During that long day, I remember hearing about something a girl had said that day: *Wouldn't it be wonderful if there was a ship with doctors and nurses that could come in after such a disaster?*

The idea stuck; I have no idea why. I remember how logical it had sounded to me. But I was as landlocked as a Colorado mountain boy could get. Young and all but clueless, I just stowed it away with all the other ideas that can fill a nineteen-year-old's head.

Soon afterwards, I recall hearing about the SS *Hope,* the world's first peacetime floating hospital. During the 1960s, the logical idea had come to life – and it captivated the world. A doctor named William Walsh was appalled by the poor health conditions he saw during his South Pacific World War II service. Dr Walsh persuaded

President Eisenhower to donate a US Navy hospital ship that he transformed with the help of donations into the SS *HOPE* ('Health Opportunities for People Everywhere').

The ship made voyages throughout the Far East, South America, and parts of Africa. I remember its simple philosophy: 'Go only where invited, and help people help themselves.' And I also remember the idealistic way it began, by asking for volunteers – drug companies to donate medicines and doctors, nurses, and technicians willing to share and teach their skills to those developing countries.

But it was not until years later, as I read Walsh's book, *A Ship Called Hope*, did memory and imagination roll together.

By that time, in the late 1970s, the SS *Hope* had been grounded after eleven successful voyages. Project Hope transformed into a land-based, developmental programme and still is working today, doing a marvellous job. At that time, there were no other nongovernmental sailing hospitals. The ocean was wide open for the Mercy Ships dream.

By the time I read Walsh's book, I was married and living in Switzerland with my wife Deyon, a nurse trained in the new field of coronary medicine. Deyon and I were young; we wanted to travel and be involved in something to make a difference with our lives. We had reconnected with Youth With A Mission, the group that had taken both of us through that hurricane, and had moved to Europe to undergo intensive language training and ultimately to direct the organisation's growing European, Middle East, and African office. But I had never forgotten my fascination with floating hospital ships. The idea still seemed incredibly viable. It had worked once; I knew it could still work. By all that is right, a citizen of the 21st century should have access to the very basics of 21st-century medical care, and I knew this could be the best and quickest way to do it.

A ship manned by experts and self-contained with its own water, power, accommodations, and medical supplies could go anywhere, and do amazing things. The problems of the developing world – lack of dependable utilities or reliable ways to deliver supplies – had always been the catch-22 of offering aid to the developing world. A ship surely could do what the best land-based or governmental organisation could do, and do it easier, quicker, and cheaper.

For months after reading Walsh's book, I couldn't stop talking about Project Hope's original floating hospital concept. In truth, though, I had been intrigued with ships ever since moving to Europe. Every chance we had to go to the Baltic port area and the Mediterranean, we would go by ferry. Living in the middle of Europe, we were surrounded by centuries of ship-going cultures. Each time we sailed somewhere, I found a way to get onto the bridge and sneak a peek into the engine room. I was fascinated with ship engines and the sheer intelligence and breadth of knowledge required to run them. A modern ship engineer has to have an understanding of petroleum, electricity generation, electronics, diesel propulsion, and sanitation and waste disposal.

I was also fascinated with the command structure. There is something about life and work onboard a ship that is sheer clarity. In the maritime world, the first rule of operation is a clear understanding of processes, systems, and structure. As a ship nears a port, a certified local pilot climbs a rope ladder and boards the ship. The pilot, who knows the local currents, shoals, and conditions, then gives orders to the captain. The pilot calls out the orders to the captain:

'Five degrees starboard!' he quietly commands.

The captain relays the command verbatim to the helmsman.

The helmsman hears the order and repeats it verbatim to make sure that the captain and the pilot know he understood correctly. And when he has brought the helm around five degrees, the helmsman repeats it again just to let the captain and pilot know he has accomplished it: 'Five degrees starboard, sir!'

That says clarity to me. Clear, crisp, and softly spoken commands bring immediate clarity and response, bring ships into port, and keep people safe. Ambiguity is dangerous – on ships or in organisations. I saw the effectiveness of clear command communication on the bridge, and it formed my future concept of the kind of 'command' structure needed for a hospital-ship effort.

Wherever we went during those years, I was drawn to the docks and to the big ships, always with a sense of wonder about why, considering I was just a Colorado farm boy. Not until years later would I find out, with delight, that my Norwegian forefathers quite likely helped to build a ship called the *Eliezer* in Norway which sailed for Sierra Leone where Mercy Ships was destined to go. Does a love for ships soak into the genes? Perhaps it does.

All I know is that while I lived in Europe, only hours from my great-grandfather's homeland, I was mesmerised with anything and everything to do with ships. At the same time I was already in a career with an established international group of volunteers who raised their own financial support for their nonprofit work. As I worked with the organisation's European, Middle Eastern, and African issues, I kept pondering new answers to old developing-world problems, hearing all the obstacles that existed for each one.

Youth has its advantages. I was naive and persistent (or stubborn, as some might say) enough to keep pondering the big questions about the developing world's problems. I truly believed there had to be streamlined, graceful answers we just weren't seeing. I was convinced that one of them had to do with the hospital-ship concept. I stored it all away, though, and went on with the work at hand.

Then our son J. P. was born.

By this time, we had two children, Heidi and Luke, both healthy and normal. But an unknown, autism-like syndrome left John Paul severely challenged, mentally and physically. What we could not know then, was that he would never be able to speak, dress, or feed himself. We loved him from the outset, but because he couldn't respond in the normal ways, we would have to learn to show our love for him through the hard work of caring for him through the years ahead.

As Deyon and I coped with the round of doctor visits and tests for our new, struggling baby, I began to wonder what we would need to provide for him. Support groups, health care, medicine, daycare centres, and education, all exist in the developed world to help the handicapped. Even our streets and buildings reflect the sensitivity for these members of our society. But that wasn't true in the rest of the world.

Even as I coped with my own emotions about my new little boy's reality, I was well aware of the enormous segments of the world's population suffering with handicaps even more severe than J. P.'s. After all, what would it be like to live in a village in Africa, or Indonesia, or Guatemala, and face a similar situation? The question now had a personal dimension. And as our fears were realised for our third child, I came face-to-face with the fundamental question about the value of a life.

And that was the moment I met Mother Teresa.

John Paul was not quite a year old when a doctor friend in India invited me to accompany him to see Mother Teresa's world-renowned work with the destitute in Calcutta. I would have a chance to see how her order, the Sisters of Charity, cared for the severely handicapped and the dying in the midst of one of the world's most impoverished cities. Her work should have been little noticed by the world, really. Yet everyone, from the most powerful leaders to everyday citizens, knew about her service to the world's forgotten, inspired by the capacity for human mercy she embodied. She had become a shining example of a person who, through dignity, honour, and respect, put words into action, 'doing' the gospel, as she so famously expressed it. Action before words – it was the same dynamic my father had expressed.

The city of Calcutta is a shock to the senses that no description can prepare you to handle. Each night, I stepped over families living on the streets, where they were born, lived, and died. I saw one water standpipe where people lined up twenty-four hours a day to pump their family's supply. Yet despite the overwhelming needy masses in Calcutta, I'd heard that Mother Teresa had instilled in her followers a gift for focusing on each individual as if he or she were the only person in the world receiving such attention and concern. And that, I was about to discover, included me.

Somehow she had learned that my one-year-old son was handicapped. I hadn't told anyone. I hadn't begun to talk about it yet; I was still finding my way. But she knew – it was the first thing she said to me. Only moments after we were introduced, Mother Teresa said something that charted the course of the rest of my life. I can hear her exact words even now: 'Your son will help you on your journey to becoming the eyes, ears, mouth, and hands for the poor.'

I was just thirty-two years old at the time. I could not have heard a more profound message.

To visit Mother Teresa was to come away changed in some meaningful way. For me, the change was, above all, the gift of clarity. The dreams and realities of my life came together in bright, meaningful focus, shining like a beacon – a ship's beacon.

All the perfectly logical reasons against the floating hospital ships concept vanished. The idea of mercy, the idea of a ship, the idea of launching a new way to bring modern medical care to all the world's citizens – it was suddenly all I could think about, talk about, dream about.

And it was what was foremost on my mind when I had dinner with a special couple one decisive Swiss night.

The Story of Reginald and Adam

Dateline: Freetown, Sierra Leone
8°30′ N 13°15′ W

They said the child's teenaged mother died from shock when she saw the disfigured face of her illegitimate 'demon baby', with a gaping hole distorting its little nose and mouth, what the modern medical world calls a cleft palette. However his mother died, the fact that the baby still lived was no less than a miracle. And that miracle came in the form of a young man – not the father, not even a relative, but a twenty-two-year-old student named Reginald.

Reginald became friends with the unmarried pregnant teenager when she left home to live with the family of the baby's young father. One morning, Reginald heard that she had gone into labour and things had gone horribly wrong. She was dead and something was wrong with the baby's face.

By Muslim tradition, the dead must be buried by sundown the same day. None of the girl's family were there to claim her body. Her adoptive mother, Dankay, away on business, would not know anything for three more days. And the baby? Forgotten in a corner. Reginald stood on the outskirts of the drama, watching, as the young father's family buried his friend and ignored the unwanted, disfigured newborn boy. With no mother to nurse him and no upper lip to suck, how could he survive? Reginald, though, knew a cleft lip was a medical problem, not a curse. He also remembered a hospital ship that offered free surgeries to fix such problems, and he had heard it was coming back. So Reginald found and convinced Dankay she could still save her daughter's child,

21

promising that he would support and care for the baby as his own son. Grandmother Dankay dried her tears and opened her heart.

Soon, the three stood expectantly in the Mercy Ships medical screening line. At three weeks old, the baby weighed just over six pounds, too weak to undergo the trauma of surgery. Nurses showed the two how to feed him formula from the lid of a baby bottle. As part of the Baby Feeding Programme, Reginald and Dankay brought the newborn faithfully to the hospital ship to check his progress. In the weeks ahead, the newborn grew stronger and rounder – and they named him Adam.

And as he grew, so did his family. Grandma Dankay cried with joy when they put Adam back into her arms after surgery, crisscrossed bandages covering his new lip. Reginald smiled the proud smile of a father and touched Adam's new face gently. And when the hospital ship left Freetown, all three watched from the dock – grandmother, father and son – no blood shared between them save the bond of love. But a family just the same.

Ship's Log: 1978

Venice, Italy
45°26′ N 12°20′ E

CHAPTER 2

THE PERFECT SHIP

One should ... be able to see things as hopeless and yet be determined to make them otherwise. – F. SCOTT FITZGERALD

Their names were Henri and Françoise André, and we had become friends after J. P.'s birth. They, too, had a handicapped son, but he had survived only a few months. So Deyon and I naturally were drawn to them. Each minute spent with J. P. after my visit to Calcutta reminded me of Mother Teresa's profound words. They were always on my mind. One day in 1978, when we were all having dinner together, I heard myself telling Henri and Françoise of my floating hospital idea. Of the one hundred largest cities in the world, more than ninety are port cities, I told them. And according to the research at the time, it was the world's port cities that also had the highest infant mortality, lowest life expectancy, and the lowest income.

'I think we're missing a simple and economical way to help change that,' I said. 'A hospital ship would do the very opposite of most ships. It would be a ship that is docked more than sailed. In fact, it would be docked most of the year, either in ports performing as a hospital ship or for maintenance, recruitment, or fund-raising. The ship wouldn't be about making a profit, so it wouldn't cost as much to operate, and another way it could be amazingly cost effective is that everyone involved would be a volunteer.

'People would pay to serve onboard a Mercy Ship,' I continued.

Henri listened politely as a friend would, and I thought that would be the end of it. But then he said, 'Why don't you come on down to the office? I'll introduce you to the man in charge of the technical side of our shipping company.'

'Your what?' I asked. I knew that Henri's family owned companies involved with commodities and grain traders, but I didn't know he had anything to do with shipping. After all, we were in landlocked Switzerland.

Henri laughed. 'The man's name is George Rouges. You can tell him about this idea.' The next thing I knew, the André shipping family had taken my crazy hospital ship dream and me under their wings. With the Swiss Atlantic expert's help, we began a feasibility study for overhauling an oceangoing vessel into a hospital ship.

Meanwhile, I began to put together a tactical deployment plan for such a ship that would sail from Europe and serve Africa. For the next year after that meeting with Henri, I spent each spare minute thinking about this hospital ship. I subscribed to shipping magazines. I kept finding ways to be invited to the bridge to talk about all things ship-wise – learning, learning, learning.

Finally, when the feasibility study seemed to show that this idea *was* actually feasible, I knew it was time to see what was available for sale. I contacted a shipping agent in London and a Cyprus friend contacted a shipping agent in the Mediterranean. Almost immediately, we received telexes listing all the ships available. About a dozen different ships potentially right for our needs were put on a spreadsheet for us to consider along with their essential facts: size, berth space, available cargo and public area space, engine type, fuel consumption per hour and day, general condition, surveying companies, the countries' flags under which they sailed, and on and on.

I began taking night trains to ports all throughout Europe to inspect ships on the market, sometimes taking my son Luke as my companion. We spent months, off and on, looking at ships, as I continued to work full time as the YWAM director for Europe, the Middle East, and Africa.

Finally, one ship from the list looked too good to be true – the *Victoria* in Venice, Italy. So this time, Deyon and I, along with a group of trusted friends and colleagues willing to support my idea, took a train to Italy to look at her.

The ship was built in 1953 by the Italian government, and owned by one of the state-owned shipping companies. It was on the market because they were modernising their fleet. She was one of three sister ships built for the legendary Lloyd Triestino luxury liner company. In the parlance of the shipping world, ships are referred to as ladies, and the female pronoun is used to describe a ship. In that context, the *Victoria* was a lovely lady, with classic shipping lines built of an era that ended after World War II because of the advent of jet air travel. She was a beautiful ship. There was midcentury elegance everywhere you looked, from her grand staircase between decks to the grand murals of hunting scenes encircling the dining rooms, to the Venetian glass lamps and wooden etchings in the meeting rooms.

But what I found out about the ship was even more fascinating, as we've met people over the years who had sailed with her in her early days. The *Victoria* was considered one of the ships on the 'ice cream route'. Upper-class citizens would take the Orient Express across to Venice, then board this fully air-conditioned ('ice cream') ship, and sail to East Africa or to colonies in Asia. In fact, a few decades earlier the word *posh* was coined to describe a voyage before air-conditioning was available: The British colonialists decided that sailing 'port out, starboard home' was the very best, coolest cabin possible. Port out, starboard home: *posh*.

The *Victoria* had sailed from Venice, Italy, through the Suez Canal, down the east coast of Africa and then across to Pakistan, India, Sri Lanka, through the Straits of Malacca and all the way up to Hong

Kong, and occasionally to Japan; then she would turn around and sail back. She was built as a passenger/cargo liner, with five cargo holds, but what made her seem even more compatible for our needs was that she was one of the few ships built during the time when every cabin had private bathroom facilities.

She seemed like our dream ship. Now we'd have to see for ourselves.

When we arrived by train over the causeway that goes out to the island of Venice, we looked out the windows of the train to behold an enormous white ship – nine decks and more than five hundred feet long. We were speechless. A team of three Italian watchmen was onboard. We climbed a rope ladder up the high side of the Italian liner and went from stem to stern, down to the double-bottom tank tops in the engine room, then up to the bridge on top. We went down again into the lower cargo holds, all five of them, climbed back up to the funnel, this time from inside the engine room, and out to the 'monkey island' area on top of the bridge. We went throughout the ship as far as we could possibly go. After inspection, this ship seemed perfect. But, we all kept thinking: *The ship is huge.*

'Shouldn't we get something smaller?' Deyon asked dubiously, as we explored the cabins designed for more than eight hundred passengers and crew.

Common sense would be to start small, wouldn't it? But I found myself thinking, *No – in fact, it might not be large enough.* The idea I was willing to give my life for, the idea that felt truly God given, was a hospital ship: actual surgeries onboard, with all the extra space that would entail for operating rooms and recovery wards. What I saw in my mind's eye as I looked around was this ship filled to its huge capacity with professionals from all walks of life bringing hope and healing to some of the most struggling parts of the world. With a ship this size, we could leave a legacy in the developing nations. *Yes,* I thought, *this ship has room enough for the whole dream.*

That was the first of many trips to see the *Victoria*. Finally, we took the next step. We needed to talk to the Italian government. The Adriatic Company officials arranged for us to fly to Rome to meet with a Mr Della Pianni, the minister of maritime affairs. We spent quite a while in the office of this Italian government minister. He asked question after question about what we had planned for the ship.

So I told him in detail about the idea of a hospital ship – a ship of mercy – sailing to offer free medical care to the developing areas of the world. His questions were very direct. It seemed he wanted to be convinced that we were not going to use it for commercial purposes. 'No,' I repeated. 'Definitely not commercial purposes; strictly humanitarian, charitable purposes only.'

His response was interesting.

'I am an old man,' he said. 'I am going to meet God myself one of these days. I, too, would like to do something to help the developing nations.' He paused a moment, then said, 'I'll sell it to you.' My heart jumped straight into my throat. Then he added, 'What are you willing to pay?'

With that sudden turn of conversation, I didn't know what to say. When I found my voice, I said, 'Scrap value?'

There are all kinds of ways to buy a ship. The cheapest way is to pay the price of the metal in it – in shipping terminology, 'scrap value'. But this ship was not ready to be scrapped. In fact, we were there at just the right time or it would have been worth far more than we'd ever have been able to pay. At that time in shipping history, a global upheaval was beginning. With the increase of air transport, the previous generation's main use of ocean liners was no longer economical. The future of the passenger shipping industry seemed gloomy.

But soon, a surprising new industry would begin. Two entrepreneurial European shipping families would very soon recreate ocean liners into today's Carnival Cruise Lines and Holland America Lines, and pioneer today's lucrative cruise industry. That meant older luxury liners would soon be at a premium; all they needed was an upgrade to be ready for a new life as a cruise ship. But that had not happened yet, so our timing was almost perfect. Any earlier, such a ship would not have been for sale; any later, it would have become a much-sought-after cruise liner.

Even with timing on our side, though, we were bidding against a Greek family-owned business whose starting offer was $2.4 million for the same ship we were hoping that the Italian government and Mr Della Pianni would sell us for scrap value.

To my surprise, he picked up the phone and called the head of the Adriatic Company in Venice. 'What is the scrap value of the *Victoria*?' he asked. We watched him nod and frown, then hang up. 'We will sell you the ship for the equivalent of the scrap value which is $1 million,' he said.

Then he asked how much time we would need to get the money. In his world, ships were bought and sold overnight. Contracts were sometimes written on napkins. Enormous amounts of money changed hands at lightning speed. I knew if we couldn't move at somewhere near lightning speed, this still could all go bust. So I told Mr Della Pianni that we needed nine months, not having any idea how long it might really take. We had enough for a deposit, but we didn't have the rest. That would take a bank. He thought a moment, then agreed. We signed a contract on July 7, 1978, and put down the deposit.

Armed with the feasibility study, financial plan, tactical plan, and a contract with the Italian government, I began visiting banks. I must have visited a dozen of them throughout Europe. No one gave me more than a few minutes of their time. The ship was worth twice the loan needed, and still I couldn't get anyone to partner with my Mercy Ships idea. Actually, I didn't blame them. What did I know about shipping? Or about hospitals, for that matter? If I had been a banker, I probably wouldn't loan money to me, either.

Finally, I went to the Union Bank of Switzerland. To my surprise, they said yes, they would make us the loan. I wouldn't find out until two decades later, while sitting by Henri André's wife, Françoise, at a Mercy Ships event, why the bank had said yes when no one else would. Henri had put in a good word on our behalf to his bank – the Union Bank of Switzerland. And he had never said a word about it to me.

So on October 5, 1978, with a million-dollar loan from a Swiss bank, the first Mercy Ship was ours. And soon it was towed by tugs to the Bay of Elevsis in Greece to begin its renovation.

What I didn't know was that it would take four years to get the ship ready to sail; four years laid up in the Mediterranean harbours; four long, struggling years that would include an oil embargo, an earthquake, and one strange, wonderful, little natural miracle.

RECRUITMENT AD

published in *Marine News and Maritime Reporter*

SHIP'S LOG: 1979–1982

Elevsis, Greece
38°2' N 23°33' E

CHAPTER 3
STRANDED IN GREECE

The way of progress is neither swift nor easy. – MARIE CURIE

The ship was ours – a ship without a crew, that is.

Immediately upon signing the contract, I began recruiting and fund-raising to transform the old luxury liner into a Mercy Ship to meet our own high expectations and the shipping industry's highest standards. We needed expert help, experts with big hearts. And we needed them fast. Not only were we going to do the upgrades needed by law, our ultimate plans included installation of three fully equipped operating rooms, a dental clinic, a laboratory, an X-ray unit, and a fifteen-hundred-ton cargo capacity. We needed deck officers, welders, plumbers, engineers, and electricians, not to mention basic staff.

I began giving lectures about the Mercy Ships idea talking about my vision to all who would listen, asking for volunteers and donations to get this first hospital ship on its way to bringing hope and healing. In hindsight, I find it almost unbelievable that we recruited any crew at all. But soon 150 people, some with families, had joined us. Our fourth child, Charles, had just been born. Deyon and I moved onboard with our children and the slowly growing team.

Thinking back, I am slightly awed by this first crew. It's one thing to join Mercy Ships now with a growing fleet of ships and years of proven service. But those who came in the early days believed in the vision of a charity hospital ship in a way that still humbles me. Soon more volunteers began trickling in. The work would start and stop, start and stop, depending on the number of volunteers onboard. As the days turned into months and the months into years, I began to worry about keeping up their enthusiasm and, quite literally, retaining their presence.

What keeps a volunteer working? A volunteer has to deeply believe in a vision and keep believing in it. The first is much easier than the latter. During those first years as the ship kept, in nautical terms, 'swinging around the anchor chain' – moving but not going anywhere – I had to remind the volunteers why they were there: 'There will be a day,' I kept saying, 'when the ship is full of crew and supplies. There will be a day when we are sailing into the needy ports of the world. There will be a day when the hospital beds will be full of those in dire need of our help.'

But that day took a very, very long time. Why did it take us so long? Because of a tactical error – I tried to save money. The ship, before it could sail, needed to be fully surveyed for $1.4 million. In other words, I could have bought the ship fully 'en class', fully surveyed, for $400,000 more than the original price. But I thought if the experts could do that for $400,000, surely with volunteer labour we could do it for less.

As they say: Penny rich, pound poor; add another year or two to your schedule. It was a novice mistake and, truthfully, it was the primary reason it took us so long. The survey turned out to be far too big a job for volunteer work. To recruit exactly the right professionals who could not only take time to volunteer but also could do the work as quickly as it needed to be done was, we found, all but impossible.

On top of that, at one stage in the repairs we were just flat out of money. And when I say we were out of money, we couldn't put fuel in the ship. If you can't put fuel in the ship to run the generators, you don't have power and you can't do repairs.

But we weren't the only ones having fuel supply problems. The first Arab oil embargo had begun and created economic chaos on a global scale. Even if we had the money, we would still have had trouble buying as much fuel as we needed.

How did we get fuel? When we bought the ship, the fuel tanks were almost full, so we began stealing from ourselves. We drained every tank so thoroughly, not a drop was left in any of them. With any small amounts of money we had, we would take fifty-five-gallon drums down to the nearest petrol station and fill them up. To make the scenario even more ridiculous, the old car we were using to drive around Greece to collect parts was a donated Mercedes post office van.

So picture it: We would load the fifty-five-gallon barrel drums into the back of that German van, drive to the nearest petrol station, and fill the drums at the pump. The Greek station owner just shook his head each time he saw us coming. I don't speak Greek, but I could imagine what he was saying: *These idiots! They don't know what they are doing. You don't fill up a ship with fifty-five-gallon drums!* But we'd fill them up, turn around, take them back to the ship, and hoist the drums up on the deck with our crane, to fuel our generators.

To give a good comparison, that would be like filling a water gun with gasoline and squirting it into your car's gas tank. But in that way, we managed to have a literal hour of power in the morning and an hour at night, to work on our renovations. During those years of painfully slow progress and low funds, we kept moving, from anchor to dry dock and back again, according to how much money we had to pay for berths.

At the same time, the economic impact of the Arab oil embargo was putting many shipping companies out of business. Already around us were older passenger liners who no longer met classification, yet were quite suitable for other uses. Every day, from our deck, we watched more ships come in to the harbour. And soon, when we were again at anchor, away from the dock, we found ourselves moored stern to bow amidst a row of ten ships.

Off to one side were four enormous crude oil tankers, clustered together with only Yokohama fenders – big rubber air balloons chained together for a cushioning effect. On the other side of us was a ship-breaking yard. It was known as the 'ship graveyard' – the last resting place before a ship is hooked on to a big cable, towed up onto the quay and taken apart by men with cutting torches. We weren't there, but we could see it all clearly from where we were anchored.

Rumours began to fly that we were in the graveyard, that the Mercy Ships idea was already a bust. We ignored them as best we could. But I confess to being more irritated by the thought that this great ship would ever be scrapped than by some personal failure. This special ship of ours had steel thicker than any ship built since that time, including the most modern cruise liner built today, the *Queen Mary II*. In other words, she was 'built like they don't build ships any more'. Even now, here in the 21st century, this same ship may never be junked. It's built too well.

But anchored in sight of the Greek ship graveyard, I also realised something potentially more serious. I knew the longer it took to set sail, the more our future would seem in doubt, and the harder it would be to inspire donations and recruit volunteers for the cause. And I saw ample evidence anchored all around us of how forces beyond one's control could vanquish dreams.

When you are that close to seeing your one truly inspired idea become real, you don't stop. When I wavered, I would run the trap lines in my mind. *Just stay the course. Keep raising funds, talk about the vision, and let the crew work.*

I'll never forget the day we finally had enough funds to fill the ship's tanks. Two small ships brought more than one thousand tons of fuel oil and slowly filled our tanks up. We watched the ship sink into the water with every ton of fuel. I was convinced I could feel the difference walking the decks. In fact, one of the tanks was a bit overfilled. We had oil running down one of the hallways on the linoleum. But nobody said a word. We were all smiles swabbing up the mess.

Finally the repairs and surveys were progressing once more and everyone seemed hopeful and upbeat again – and that was the moment that the earthquake hit.

The Bay of Elevsis where we were, just southwest of Athens, is known for its calm waters. Picture a Mediterranean setting – that would be it. So we were surprised to say the very least. The first quake hit after 10 p.m. We had turned off the generators and all was quiet. Suddenly the ship rolled and creaked and groaned. And when I say, *roll*, I mean a rather significant roll to an uncomfortable angle. At the time, 175 of us were living onboard. I think every one of us went topside to peer over the railing, expecting to see where another ship had hit us during the night. But we saw nothing, so we all went back to our cabins.

Then, at about 5 a.m., our second officer decided to go topside on his watch. He was standing on the deck when the second major seismic shock hit. He heard people screaming on the island of Salamina, about a mile off our stern; their buildings were crumbling. He literally watched the quake come towards us – the earth moved, then the water moved, then the ship moved. We knew then it was an earthquake. So, we responded immediately. We'd already begun to store donations such as blankets, clothing, and water for future relief work. And so when the earthquake hit all around us, we were ready to help. We moved alongside the dock, offloaded the goods into vans, and began distribution to those in need.

That Greek earthquake, happening all around us, turned out to be our first disaster relief effort, undertaken before we were even up and running. The earthquake also shook us up in ways we could never have guessed at the time. We were soon to have another lesson in how big the world was and how full of surprises it could be. It came in the form of fish.

After the earthquake, we once more found ourselves without power. We lost permission from the Greek authorities to live onboard during the refurbishing, so our new crew and their families were forced to move onshore. And where did we move? Into a hotel complex condemned because of the earthquake. Actually, it was a lovely beach hotel complex with bungalows only a short distance from the ship. Even though some of the bungalows where we stayed had been slightly affected by the quake, they seemed safe. As long as we stayed away from the condemned area, so were we.

The owners were glad to have us while they contemplated their renovation woes. Every day the crew and I went back and forth to the ship by launch, which was often an experience itself. Our Greek port was a protected harbour, but it had its share of three- to four-foot swells that made getting from the launch to the gangway of the ship an athletic event at times. But the bungalows were right on the water, and everybody enjoyed the beach.

One early morning, one of our volunteers was doing just that. Only a few other people, mainly native Greeks, were around. Suddenly, as they all were having a nice moment communing with nature, fish started to jump out of the sea.

Rushing back to the bungalows, the volunteer began telling everyone in sight to grab any available container. As we were financially strapped, this was a bonanza and she knew it. So she and everyone at the bungalows with a bucket joined the Greeks on the beach who were already gathering up fish.

Then, as quickly as it happened, it stopped. By all accounts, that was the only place it happened.

The fish were of the herring family, from five to twelve inches in length. For natives of Scandinavia, this fish was well known as a delicacy. We had about thirty Scandinavian members of the crew at the time, and they were ecstatic. Our Norwegian chef prepared the fish in a special Norwegian way, and everybody enjoyed ultra-fresh fish, straight from the Mediterranean Sea.

Two to three days later, at about 8 a.m., I was meeting on our little bus with the technical and navigation crew, before they took the launch to the ship. Suddenly, my wife Deyon appeared, exclaiming: 'The fish are jumping out of the sea again!'

Well, I don't care how important your meeting is. You can't continue a meeting when something like that is happening. I had fished some prime river areas as a Colorado mountain boy with feet planted on *terra firma,* but rarely had I caught more than a few fish in an entire day. So I bailed out of that bus. This I had to see!

There they were again: Fish were beaching themselves by the thousands. So, for the next several hours, we all collected as many fish as we could. We collected them in plastic bags. We collected them in tubs and buckets. We even collected them in wheelbarrows borrowed from the hotel. We used everything available. When we brought them back to the outside kitchen area around the hotel pool, we put them on a stainless steel table to clean and preserve them, putting them in groups of tens, then fifties, then hundreds. Ultimately we counted 8,301 fish – almost two tons worth.

The other people on the beach, several Greek families, who had experienced this phenomenon with us, were just as awed as we were. None of them had ever seen anything like it, they told us. So as they took their own fish bonanza home with them, the word spread quickly. No doubt our Scandinavian crew also talked about it up and down the wharf, especially about how our chef prepared them.

The next thing we knew, a Greek television company arrived, cameras and reporters from a show as famous in Greece as CNN's *Larry King Live* in the English-speaking world.

'We understand that the fish jumped out of the sea for you,' one of them said, and they wanted to know how we made this happen.

'We didn't have anything to do with it,' we said, then asked them to explain it to us.

But because of the nature of their business, the television reporters made a sensational story of it, no doubt for prime time. The story spread like wildfire, and even though Greek locals were all around us when it happened, somehow we got all the credit because it happened on the beach where we were staying.

Months later, just before we finally were ready to set sail, a local shipping company sponsored a reception for us at the Athens Yacht Club, where all the major Greek ship owners were members. There I met the man, for instance, who had bid against us for the *Victoria*. He told me that he had bought a ship in Latin America and was about to completely outfit it. Then, on the spot, he offered us a million dollars in cash to swap ships with him. That, for me, was confirmation of a choice well made in buying the *Victoria*.

So, here we were with all these well-known ship owners who were on the same level as Aristotle Onassis and who were attending the reception because they were fascinated with our use of an old passenger liner for humanitarian purposes. And what did they all ask us to bring? Our chef's hors d'oeuvres made with the fish that had jumped out of the sea.

Whatever it was, the fish phenomenon had been amazing. Even the Greeks thought so. Looking back, I know only two things for certain about the experience: The fish were delicious, and the thrill of seeing such an occurrence was one of the strangest and most remarkable moments of my life.

I had no way of knowing, at the time, that I had not heard the last of that remarkable event.

On July 7, 1982, we were ready to sail. We christened our ship the

Anastasis, the Greek word for 'resurrection', a fitting name on many levels after all the years it took to get this far. That day, sailing from the Bay of Elevsis, was unforgettable. The Blue Peter Flag was hoisted, signifying the ship would sail in twenty-four hours. The last finishing touches had been applied, and our new logo, a figure carrying a torch across a globe, was riding high on our ship's funnel. We were on our way. Tugboats pulled alongside and slowly inched us away from our berth. Everyone was on deck. The ship was alive again and headed to the open sea.

We were bound for our first stop, the island of Malta. At Malta's port of Valetta, we did a nice 'Mediterranean mooring', parking the ship with the stern in and the anchors down, the captain allowing the stern to swing around – as if we had backed in.

Why did we stop? We were flying a Maltese flag.

And why had we chosen Malta's flag to fly?

Beyond the professional and nautical benefits offered with the registry, we had a special feeling for the flag itself. The Maltese flag displays the Maltese cross, a cross that was developed by the knights of St John, who were called the Hospitallers. During the Middle Ages, they developed what they called 'hospices' throughout the Middle East where they would care for weary and sick travellers. It seemed the perfect flag for the very first Mercy Ship. As the ship left Malta, one of our crew pulled out his trumpet and played a salute from the stern.

At long last, the Mercy Ship *Anastasis* was sailing into the world.

THE STORY OF MARIAMA AND ANSU

 Dateline: Freetown, Sierra Leone
8°30' N 13°15' W

Mariama heard shots in the distance as she put her baby Ansu on
her back.

'Run!' shouted Mariama's husband, Lahem, as he grabbed their four
other children and headed into the Sierra Leone streets. Rapid gunfire
drowned out the screams of people being hit by flying bullets and
exploding grenades from rebel soldiers. The country's civil war had
returned to their village. Mariama watched as Lahem herded their
other children ahead of him. Suddenly, a surprised look came over his
face. He crumpled to the ground, dead. The rebels simply advanced
over the bodies, moving closer. She had no time for goodbyes. Two of her
children had already been killed in an earlier attack. Their only hope
lay in reaching the nearby jungle.

Only when they stopped long enough to catch their breath did
Mariama feel the blood soaking the left side of her dress, coming
from little Ansu on her back. His left knee, shattered by fragments
of the grenade that killed his father, made his leg hang at an odd
angle. Mariama bound it as best she could by ripping her skirt
into strips.

For weeks, Mariama and her five children wandered through the
jungles, feeding on bush yams and ground nuts, drinking from streams,
gathering rice left on the ground of small farms. Eventually they came
to a town where they and others were transported by a nongovernmental organisation to a camp 200 miles away.

Ten years later Mariama returned to her hometown of Mobai where she provided for her family by practising her midwifery skills. Her son Ansu, now twelve years old, had spent his life crippled because of his shattered knee.

One day, Mariama learned of the hospital ship screening in a nearby village. Could the hospital ship help her poor boy? They went to see. When Ansu's time in the long screening line came, the doctor smiled and handed Ansu an appointment card for surgery onboard the ship in Freetown. Within days, not only had Ansu received surgery on his knee, but Mercy Ships' New Steps programme had fitted him with calipers and provided physical therapy to strengthen his legs.

Mother and son spent the next few weeks in the ship's recovery ward. Finally, she said, after her long story of terror and death and despair, she felt a peace she'd long forgotten. And Ansu? He was learning how to walk for the first time in his life.

SHIP'S LOG: 1982–1984

Champerico, Guatemala
14°30' N 91°92' W

Auckland, New Zealand
36°44' S 174°50' E

Honolulu, Hawaii
21°18' N 157°5' W

CHAPTER 4
LAUNCHED!

God, grant me the serenity to accept the things I cannot change, the courage to change the things I can, and the wisdom to know the difference. – REINHOLD NIEBUHR

I remember that first sail across the wide, open sea – the pleasure of that voyage after all those years at anchor. For twenty-one gloriously beautiful days, we sailed across a smooth Atlantic Ocean watching porpoises and dolphins playing at the bow, while we moved through the Panama Canal to dock in Los Angeles.

During our time in Greece, we had decided to bring the ship to the United States where we planned to open a resource and support office to raise funds and recruit volunteers from the United States' pool of talent. We hoped to inspire the same fervour that had fuelled the SS *Hope*'s volunteers a generation earlier. We already had an office in Switzerland that we hoped would be the first in a long line of resource offices worldwide.

Meanwhile, we would also perform our first official relief effort. The Ixil Indians in Guatemala had been the victims of civil war two years in a row. Their crops had been destroyed one year by the government's troops and the next year by the insurgent troops. We decided to help.

In the port of Los Angeles, thousands of visitors, including the media, toured the Mercy Ship. We announced our relief effort plans and soon the donations poured in. That first cargo consisted of twenty tons of cornmeal, one hundred thousand dollars' worth of seeds for crops, twenty-three thousand new shirts, enough steel roofing for 750 homes, hand tools and farm equipment, generators, a portable sawmill, medical supplies, and a mobile dental facility. Local longshoremen donated their services, volunteering to load cargo for two solid days, free of all charges. With the total value of seeds and high-quality gifts in kind, the value of our cargo for our first official relief voyage was equivalent to a million dollars – the exact purchase amount of the ship itself.

As soon as we were loaded, we headed for the Guatemalan port of Champerico. Because the ship was too big for the dock, we anchored offshore and were carried ashore literally like big, breathing bunches of bananas. The sea village was an old banana loading port. In fact, the crane used to haul us to the dock was actually steam driven.

The banana barges were brought out to the ship and tied alongside. Our crew had to ease into a cargo net 'sling' with thick plywood in the bottom, stand squashed together, while a crane lowered this netted cargo of humans over the side of the ship and into the barge where everyone wiggled out of the net to be motored ashore. Then everyone had to step back into the nets to be lifted up to the pier by the steam-engine crane. Adding in to the equation the rolling four-foot swells, we knew we were in for an adventure before we even set foot on land. As you might imagine, it took us quite a while to unload.

After our experience in Guatemala, we responded to calls for help in the South Pacific where deadly cyclones that made worldwide news had almost decimated Fiji and Tonga. We planned to sail to New Zealand to pick up a small load of donated supplies waiting for us, with hopes that our presence could help generate more.

We didn't have to wait long. Shortly after arriving in New Zealand, I received a call from the country's governor general, Sir David Beatty: 'New Zealand would like to respond to this devastation in Fiji and Tonga, I would like to use my office to start

Operation Good Samaritan. We will fill up your ship with building lumber from our mills and with corrugated iron for tin roofs. We have also just trained firefighters in several of the affected cities, so we want to donate six fire engines and will help put them on your deck . . .' The governor general went on and on, detailing this huge plan for us.

Finally, I said, 'Sir David, you don't know anything about us.'

He said, 'Oh yes, I do, Don. I was in Washington, DC, last year and I sat at a dinner table with a couple from Switzerland – Henri and Françoise André. I think you know them.'

The Andrés, again. Our guardian angels.

In the next few days, we sailed to fifteen different ports in New Zealand, filling our holds with relief material for the islands.

While in New Zealand, I had another interesting phone call. An American business acquaintance wanted to donate a coastal cruise ship he'd just bought to help the Mercy Ships cause. The ship was a fraction of the size of the *Anastasis*, but it had a shallow draft, only twelve feet, which would allow her to operate in areas such as the Guatemalan port we'd just left without worrying about banana barges and cargo nets for transport onto land. And we had no more said 'thank you' and began brainstorming how to pay for the needed refurbishing than the Canadian government chartered it back as a temporary replacement for a former fleet mate, and paid us enough money to cover almost all the modifications.

So in the spring of 1985, an entirely new crew was recruited for the new ship that was destined to begin a Caribbean Mercy Ships effort. The ship was rechristened *Good Samaritan*, but to her crew throughout the next few years she was affectionately known as the 'Little Giant'. By November, the newest Mercy Ship departed on her inaugural voyage from Jacksonville, Florida, bound for Haiti, the poorest country in the Western Hemisphere.

Back in New Zealand, we were now ready to sail, our holds full with not only our original goods, but also the governor general's goodwill operation donations, including the six fire engines on our deck. So we set sail on the Pacific Ocean. By its very name, we expected calm, 'pacific' waters. Let me tell you – they weren't. We found ourselves in one of the worst storms since the cyclones had hit the very islands we were trying to help. Two-thirds of the crew were either prone, face downwards, on the floor or flat on their backs from sea sickness. During this storm, the sea spray shorted the electrical circuit on one of the big fire trucks we had lashed to the deck. Not only was everyone sicker than sea dogs with the roiling ocean, but a fire engine siren was blowing in the background.

During such a storm, what seamen call a 'rogue wave' can hit a ship. You can feel it hit; the whole ship shudders with the power of that one wave. Normally, to be hit by a rogue wave is not a good thing, but this time was an exception. Finally, after what seemed like hours of listening to that siren, a rogue wave slammed into the ship, hitting the deck so hard that its saltwater spray short-circuited the siren.

We survived the storm to sail and offload the relief materials without a hitch. Our original plans after New Zealand were to visit Papua New Guinea, then sail on to Asia and Hong Kong, taking medical and relief donations as we could and making contacts for the future. But first, we were scheduled for a stop in Hawaii. We'd been asked to deliver cargo to help a needy Youth With A Mission project. While we were sailing between islands, something happened that turned us the opposite direction, stranding us again, but at the same time charting a course into another future.

The United States Coast Guard boarded the ship for what should have been a routine inspection of a foreign-registered vessel calling at an American port. Although there had been no previous trouble at any of the thirty ports that the *Anastasis* had already visited, including a harbour in the United States, this time would be different. We were fully certified with Lloyd's Register, completely seaworthy and safe, but Lloyds had classified our ship as a cargo vessel. We weren't really a cargo ship, but we weren't a passenger ship, either. We had onboard 337 people including twenty married couples and more than fifty children, representing twenty-five nationalities. While they weren't cargo, they weren't passengers, either. There simply wasn't a classification for what we were.

We had come in to American waters, with property certification as a cargo vessel, and now the authorities had decided we were a passenger ship. We had heat detectors. What we didn't have was a sprinkler system, and according to International Safety of Life at Sea (SOLAS) standards, a passenger ship must have one. That might sound like a small thing to add. But on a ship the size of the *Anastasis* that would include retrofitting several miles of steel pipe and sprinkler heads at the cost of a million dollars.

After all the years in Greece, this was quite a blow. We had a choice: We could lift the anchors and sail straight to Hong Kong and never return to US waters, or we could do whatever the US authorities wanted us to do. But really, there was no choice. Once a shadow is cast over how you operate a ship, you'll always have a problem. For the sake of the hospital ship future we still believed in so deeply, we decided to comply.

We pulled into Honolulu, set anchor, and moved all the families ashore to live in three different campgrounds while we began upgrading to meet the SOLAS standards. Eighteen months passed before we headed to sea again towards British Columbia to complete the final modifications required to gain passenger certification.

And in the midst of it all, I received the strangest call of my life.

THE STORY OF DAISY

Excerpted from *Mercy Ships News*, Asian Edition, Spring 2000

Dateline: Pulupandan, Philippines
10°31' N 122°48' E

Hiding behind oversized sunglasses, Daisy shyly entered the orthopaedic screening exam room. With her mother by her side, the twenty-year-old waited quietly while Mercy Ships orthopaedic surgeon Dr Tim Browne examined her arms and legs. Finding no orthopaedic problems, Dr Browne asked her to remove the dark glasses that concealed her eyes. Shocked, he looked into the disfigured face of the young woman. Scars from a botched cleft palate surgery she had received as a child distorted her lower eyelids, turning them down and under. Daisy could not close her eyes.

Dr Browne felt instant compassion for her but without an ophthalmologist trained in plastic surgery, a rare combination, there was little the Caribbean Mercy crew could do to help her.

So Dr Browne referred Daisy to the Mercy Ships optical screening clinic, hoping that at least she could receive a new pair of glasses for her failing eyesight. There she was examined and asked to return the following week.

Meanwhile, Dr Rafael Rodriguez, an ophthalmologist from Manila, had arrived to volunteer with the ship's floating eye surgery hospital for a few days. When the ophthalmologist examined Daisy, everyone was in for a surprise. What no one on the Caribbean Mercy knew was that Dr Rodriguez was trained in ophthalmic plastic surgery, precisely the kind of surgery Daisy needed.

Daisy, though, would need to travel to Manila for the surgery, where

Dr Rodriguez could arrange to do the reconstructive procedure. Other friends of Mercy Ships, Congressman Chnalrie Cojuango and his wife, Vice Mayor Rio, volunteered to sponsor Daisy's flight to Manila.

Skin grafts from behind Daisy's ears were used to patch the facial area, restoring her eyes to normal shape. For the first time in her life, Daisy was able to close her tired eyes.

Back home, recovered fully, Daisy discovered a normal life waiting for her, with the wonder of eyes that close and a face she can show to the world.

SHIP'S LOG: 1984–1986

Athens, Greece
37°58' N 23°43' E

CHAPTER 5

ON TRIAL IN GREECE

All the great things are simple, and many can be expressed in a single word: freedom; justice; honour; duty; hope; mercy.

— SIR WINSTON CHURCHILL

Almost three years after we had sailed from Greece, as the *Anastasis* sat in yet another bay 'swinging around our anchor chain', I received a shore-to-ship phone call from Costas Macris, a friend in Athens, informing me that my name appeared on a docket along with his in an Athens court.

To say I was shocked is an enormous understatement, not only for myself, but also for Costas.

Costas Macris was from a well-known family in Greece. His uncle was a sculptor famous enough to have his work prominently placed in the Athens Museum of Modern Sculpture. A Presbyterian pastor, Costas had befriended us while we worked to make the *Anastasis* seaworthy.

The rest of his words sank in very slowly: Also on the docket was the name of another crew leader onboard, Alan Williams, a British citizen from New Zealand. The Greek authorities had not even bothered to notify us. Costas told me that I'd be involved in the trial 'in absentia', so there was nothing to worry about. He told me he was requesting a delay in the trial. As non-Greek citizens, we didn't have to return to stand trial, but as a Greek, he did. The question that hung in the air as we talked was obvious: Would I consider returning to Athens, bringing Alan with me? Otherwise, Costas would stand trial alone.

And if I wasn't shocked before, I was certainly shocked to hear the charges – proselytism and attempted psychological abduction of a minor. Costas explained that the charges were being brought by the mother of a young man named Kostas Kotopoulos. I remembered the teenager. We met both the father and son while doing earthquake relief work. His parents were divorced, and the boy was living with his father. I remembered his father telling some of our group how his son was 'mesmerised' by the ship.

'My son really wants to learn English and he likes playing with your children. Do you mind if I bring him to the ship from time to time?' the father had asked. The boy was about the same age as my daughter and some of the other children. We could see that he was incredibly bright and curious. Sure, we had told the father. His son could visit anytime.

As for my friend Costas Macris, he was well known in Greece for another interesting accomplishment. He had taken the *Living Bible*, which was a worldwide phenomenon at the time, and translated parts of it into modern Greek. Controversy accompanied the whole idea of a Bible in modern vernacular, but most Christians around the world embraced it, especially young people. Macris's modern Greek *Living Bible* was a best-seller in the country in the early eighties. So Macris was well known, his family was well known, but what I didn't know was, *we* were well known. We weren't well known because of the earthquake relief effort; it was because of the fish jumping from the sea.

I was intrigued to learn that a surprising number of Greek citizens still recalled the television coverage of that fish event, but not in an accurate way. The Greek television crew had made the fish story about us, not the remarkable fish phenomenon. We were the ship and crew that had sailed into port and made the fish jump from the sea. I tried to put myself in the mother's shoes. With all that dramatic and memorable press coverage, did she begin to wonder about this 'strange' foreign ship and crew's effect on her son? Perhaps. Considering that the son in question was now nineteen, an adult under Greek law, and currently working in his father's business, why did it matter? The ship and her crew were now half a world away; two years had passed. Greece, to me, was already a fading memory.

I could only assume that was the psychological abduction part of the accusation. The proselytising charge somehow must have been related to Costas Macris's Greek translation of the *Living Bible* and the box of them he had given us for the earthquake relief work – plus the fact that we were not Greek Orthodox, the state-funded religion of Greece.

Accusations of proselytism were a real problem in Greece. They had become an almost common occurrence. Greece, with its incredibly rich and complex history, had laws still on the books meant to protect the state church, and therefore protect the Greek way of life and faith. That was especially the case during the early 20th century, when Greece was re-establishing its national independence after centuries of Muslim rule.

Of course, we didn't know much of this, so we took this charge very badly. Mercy Ships had crew and volunteers from every walk of life. We were learning daily that cultural respect was part of such diversity. Although Mercy Ships' values were deeply rooted in the Christian faith, my growing vision, especially after meeting Mother Teresa, was that we were going to be more about love in action, less about words, similar to other charities such as the Salvation Army.

I realised early on that if we allowed medicine to become the heart of the ship, then every port in the world would open to us. If not, many doors would close and the poorest of the poor would never be able to receive what we alone might be able to offer them. So I considered the situation carefully, turning it over in my mind. From my viewpoint, no one onboard was trying to change the boy's religion. After all, he was already a Greek Orthodox Christian. The boy we met, whose father asked if he could spend time with us on the ship to practise his English and hang out with our kids, was a teenager with the normal teenage issues who seemed also rather lonely, as many teenagers of divorce are. Our crew clearly recalled giving a copy of Costas's translated *Living Bible* to comfort and encourage the boy in the same spirit we handed out copies during the recent earthquake relief work.

Even though I had lived in a Greek harbour for three years, I was beginning to realise how little I understood the country's culture or its laws. I just knew the charges weren't true. As an American reared to believe that freedom to choose one's own religion was a basic human right, I also fought a feeling of outrage at the whole situation.

But most of all, I worried about my friend who wanted to clear his name so much that he'd go to court over such a strange accusation; my friend who did not expect me to come back.

So why could I not quit wondering if I should?

To go back made no sense on almost every level. I had a family to support, not to mention a fledgling organisation that was struggling to fulfil its true potential. 'In absentia' all but states the expectations of a 'no-show'. The fact that neither of us had been notified also spoke volumes. I didn't want to be naive about it. I had heard enough stories about the absence of justice in political systems around the world to know that anything was a possibility. But I couldn't stop thinking about Greece and about Costas Macris.

So I found myself discussing this at Thanksgiving a few weeks later with my brother, sister, and parents. Mercy Ships was once again at a critical stage, I pointed out. I was American, not Greek. These were not my laws, so, wasn't this really a matter between

Costas and his country's legal system? After all, what would happen to my family if I went to jail because of the lack of religious freedom in another nation? And not just any nation, but a nation considered the very cradle of democracy? It made no sense from any angle.

After a few minutes, my dad said, 'Son, I don't know why we are even discussing this.'

'Why is that, Dad?' I asked.

'Because I have always taught you to do what is right, and what is right is that you go back and stand with that friend of yours who *is* Greek and doesn't have the luxury you do of choosing whether to face this crisis or not.'

Dad summarised what was bothering me.

For Costas, a guilty verdict would damage his reputation, at best; at worst, he could actually see prison time for things the rest of us hold so dear – justice and religious freedom. The least I could do for Costas Macris, who had helped Mercy Ships during our slow, slow years in Greece, was to go back and testify on his behalf. As it turned out, Alan had come to the same conclusion.

That's when the surprises began!

To the surprise of everyone, we made plans to return.

To the surprise of the Greek authorities, we showed up and testified at the trial.

To our surprise, we were all found guilty.

But the guilty verdict wasn't a surprise to the Greeks. Proselytism accusations were so common that some attorneys actually specialised in them. Our next attorney, a Catholic, had represented more proselytism cases than any other attorney in the country – the problem was he hadn't won a single one, nor had anyone, to my knowledge. The abuse of proselytism laws was one of Greece's major problems of the day, a court system dealing with old laws creating damaging prejudice that was playing out much like our racial prejudice in the United States, but this prejudice was playing out along cultural lines. For instance, we soon learned that neither Protestants nor Catholics could be schoolteachers or officers in the Greek army.

Long-held social lines were being tested here just as they were around the world. And Costas, Alan, and I had been caught in the middle.

After being found guilty, we were sentenced to three and a half years.

I thought we would go straight to jail. Instead, the appeal process began on the spot. We surrendered our passports for documentation, and to our surprise, the judge returned them immediately. He said Alan and I were free to go, but that we would be added to the docket of the appellate court schedule. Then the judge made it crystal clear that if the appellate court upheld the lower court's finding, we would have only one more appeal, and that would be to the Greek Supreme Court. But – and this was a *big* but – if we were found guilty at the appellate court level, we would go straight to jail.

Think about it. We were handed back our passports, told to go home and come back in eighteen months for another trial that, if we lost, would mean we'd go straight to prison. That told me that the Greek authorities wanted us to stay this time 'in absentia'.

But of course, we again went back. The decision, this time, wasn't as easy or as quick in coming. Deyon and I went through the process of adding three and a half years to the ages of each of our kids. That was an eye-opener. Was this foolhardy? Again, what about Mercy Ships? We had two ships and about 350 staff by that time. Wasn't that more important? Would this still be 'doing the right thing' as my father had first said? A prison sentence is as real as a reality check gets. After all, just because it was right in one instance didn't mean it was automatically right in the next.

And yet Alan and I decided we should go back.

But this time, we were prepared.

When Alan and I left Greece after the first trial, we went straight home and contacted both the British and the US embassies. We mounted a massive public relations campaign, produced a mound of petitions signed and delivered to the Greek embassies in Washington and every Western European nation. More than four hundred thousand Americans alone signed petitions to Greek Prime Minister Papandreou. US congressmen sent letters to the Greek government. California Governor Deukmejian wrote Greek President Sartzetakis and so did President Ronald Reagan.

The argument went something like this: How is this possible? Greece is a signatory to the United Nations Declaration of Human Rights, and one of the most basic rights is the freedom to choose one's own faith without penalty. How could that not be an option in the nation that considers itself the birthplace of the democratic system?

Soon we learned that others in Greece began to see this case as one that could help change these outmoded laws to more accurately reflect the modern Greek thinking. We suddenly realised we were becoming involved in something bigger than ourselves, and in a detached, intellectual way, I became fascinated with what I was learning about international justice and human rights. With Mercy Ships always on my mind, especially as I contemplated its future, as well as my own, I couldn't help, even then, to see how the same sort of injustices might play out in the developing world.

On May 21, my wife's fortieth birthday, the court case began in Athens. Alan and I, along with Deyon and two of our children, flew back to Greece to join Costas Macris before the three-judge panel sat to decide the case.

The witnesses for our defence began lining up. A former director of studies at the International Institute of Human Rights in Strasbourg, France, testified as an expert on human rights. The

International Commission of Jurists sent an observer to ensure that the human rights of the defendants were upheld.

The daughter of a former prime minister, a professor of law at Athens University, testified on our behalf and so did two Greek Orthodox priests. One of the priests said, 'These non-orthodox were the first ones to respond after our earthquake, bringing blankets and clothing and food and potable water. We have partnered with them; we know these people are not like they are made out to be.'

'This is not even an issue with the Orthodox church,' the other said. 'This has been politicised. Costas Macris was only doing what the church is supposed to do for its youth.'

Amazingly enough, even the Greek public prosecutor told the judges that, in his opinion, the state had made a mistake in prosecuting the case, since it was neither factually nor legally true.

The verdict from the three-judge panel came quickly just after midnight on the fifth day of the trial: Not guilty. We were free to go and Costas's name had been cleared. After this case, I was told that the laws began to slowly change, that Greeks of all faiths soon were able to become army officers and teachers. I was also told that if we had lost, the case would have gone to the European Court of Human Rights. The legal arguments opposing the Greek anti-proselytising law were used in other cases.

On a personal level, it would take me years to process what happened. While justice did ultimately prevail for me, I went home resolved to understand what justice really meant in the context of everyday work and life. In the years to come, as we moved forward with Mercy Ships, I became determined to root all our efforts in a deep sense of justice – physically, economically, emotionally, spiritually, and legally.

There's another chapter to the story, by the way. A few years after the trial, the boy involved – Kostas – contacted us. By that time, he was even more multilingual, eventually becoming fluent in five languages and earning two graduate degrees abroad. He had recently found himself thinking again and again about the Mercy Ship he'd visited so often as a boy. That was why he had called. He asked me for a job, then and there. With his linguistic and developmental skills, not to mention the drama of our lives intertwining, how could I say no? All these years later, he's still with us.

I CAN SEE!

Excerpted from *Mercy Ships Newsletter*, North American edition, Summer 1987

 Dateline: February 17, 1987
17°53' N 102°12' W Lazaro Cardenas, Mexico

Señora Refugio Camacho shuffled up the gangway, her daughter hovering by her side, the rolling and rocking of the ship feeling, no doubt, like the recent earthquake. The ship's crew gathered near the gangway, wanting to catch a glimpse of their first surgery patient.

She was sixty-eight years old, face lined, grey wisps of hair escaping from her bun, hands calloused and arthritic, eyes dull with fading years and cloudy with cataracts. And she was stepping into a strange world, a big hospital ship that had anchored near her home after the Mexico earthquake.

With a red ink thumbprint, she signed the patient consent form, donned a yellow paper gown and surgical cap, and with a final shaky smile at her daughter's retreating touch, she was led into surgery. An assortment of medical professionals from Mexico and around the world who had arrived after Mercy Ships put out a call for expert help, all crowded into the room for this history in the making as Dr Bob Dyer performed the cataract surgery.

And that was also the scene the next morning as well, as everyone excitedly gathered around Señora Camacho to watch Dr Dyer carefully remove the eye patch. As the first eye patch fell away, Señora Camacho looked towards her daughter and gasped, 'Yo puedo ver! Yo puedo ver!' I can see! I can see! She grabbed Dr Dyer's hand, 'Gracias! Gracias!'

The Mercy Ship was now, finally, a hospital ship.

SHIP'S LOG: 1986–1987

Lazaro Cardenas, Mexico
17°5' N 102°12' W

CHAPTER 6

A True Hospital Ship

Whoever is spared personal pain must feel himself called to help in diminishing the pain of others. – ALBERT SCHWEITZER

When I returned from Greece, I came back ready to see Mercy Ships finally become what I'd first envisioned so long ago. Before Hawaii, I had allowed the hospital ship vision, the idea that came into clear-eyed focus after meeting Mother Teresa, to be postponed by calls for relief work, all worthy efforts but not my original vision. Being a relief ship was a marvellous thing, but I knew others could do that. In my heart, the dream I was willing to give my life for was the dream of a fleet of hospital ships.

That was what was on my mind when I heard about the Mexico City earthquake only weeks after my return. The passenger upgrades almost finished, the *Anastasis* was now in British Columbia finishing the last bits of work to gain the SOLAS certification. It would soon be time to sail again. So I went to Mexico to investigate an invitation by the provincial government to bring the Mercy Ship to a coastal area called Lazaro Cardenas, overlooked by other relief organisations centred on Mexico City. I flew into the port city of Acapulco to see what we might do. And that's where the *Anastasis* first became a true hospital ship.

I drove north to Lazaro Cardenas, the on-land site nearest the earthquake epicentre just offshore. Houses were down everywhere, grain elevators damaged, buildings crushed, and the hospital for the poor built by the Swiss government several years earlier had been severely damaged. First-aid treatment was obviously needed, but so was every sort of medical treatment, including surgery. Our medical team was already working in the town's general hospital, which was available for patients who could afford to pay for their medical services. One of our first medical volunteers, a California surgeon named Dr Gary Parker, had already performed cleft lip and palate operations, a type of surgery previously unavailable yet desperately needed in that rural area.

'Isn't there anything you can do?' someone asked.

Yes, I remember thinking.

It was time.

The ship's holds were already filled with more than $2 million in relief goods including a $100,000 fire truck and, on a subsequent voyage, an ambulance, and thousands of dollars' worth of medical equipment, including a hospital X-ray machine and dental equipment. And now, the Mercy Ship was also equipped with a new eye-surgery clinic. So while the volunteer crew built shelters and ran health clinics on land, the medical team set up screenings for the first surgeries. The *Anastasis* was about to become a fully functioning hospital ship. Medical care would no longer be an afterthought of the charity; it was going to be the primary focus – starting now.

When the government officials heard what I thought the *Anastasis* was capable of doing, they began broadcasting from the state-controlled radio stations about the Mercy Ship coming their way – letting their people know we were ready, willing, and able to do free surgeries. They only had to come. And they did.

Can you imagine how they must have felt, trusting their health to strangers on a ship? Suffering makes you brave, I believe. And the very bravest, the very first patient, was Señora Refugio Camacho, a sixty-eight-year-old woman, eyes cloudy with cataracts, hobbling along on the arm of her daughter. The team who were on hand to help Dr Bob Dyer was a fittingly international one – a local Mexican anaesthesiologist, a surgical nurse from South Africa, doctors from New Zealand and California, as well as a remarkable New Zealand woman named Simonne McCluskey who would eventually marry the eye surgeon and become my replacement as the *Anastasis'* executive director. The next morning, I don't mind admitting that tears came to my eyes when Señora Camacho grabbed Dr Dyer's hand and said: 'Yo puedo ver!'

I can see!

In the following weeks, patients from babies to great-grandmothers came onboard the big hospital ship sightless, and left seeing the world in all its glory. From cataract removal to crossed-eye corrections, the medical team gave the gift of sight to them all. None of us ever tired of witnessing those first hesitant moments as the bandages come off and the patient's brain begins to process the gift of sight.

When I think back, though, one special story does come to mind. We had a family travel to find us – the Tellez family. The couple had twelve children; four who were blind from birth because of congenital cataracts. When Señor Tellez heard the government's radio announcement of free eye surgeries, he put his four blind children in a little motorised dugout canoe and travelled down the Rio Balsas to Lazaro Cardenas. Then he led his children out of the canoe onto a public bus and made his way to the port, leading them all up the ship's gangway. They were a sight to behold. This is the image I will forever see: The children, from eldest to youngest lined up behind the other, hand to hand, Señor Tellez in the lead, all in step, slowly making their way onto the Mercy Ship.

But as fascinating as that image was, nothing can compare to watching a child see for the very first time. I had the privilege of witnessing it on that day and on many days since. We take our sight so much for granted that it's hard to grasp how amazing the moment is when the brain signals the miracle of sight. For those like the Tellez children, born blind with cataracts, the optic nerve has never been damaged. But since this is the first time in their lives their brains have been called on to translate images through their eyes, the process does not happen instantly. And if you're privileged to witness such a drama, you notice the same distinct, dramatic pause as the brain registers the incoming images for the first time. You first see it in their faces – the surprise, the joy, the wonder – and then, finally, you see it in their eyes.

And when the patient is a child, the next few seconds are even more unforgettable. Bandages are removed from the child's eyes and immediately the eyes begin to search for the child's mother. Every blind child knows his or her mother by the sound of her voice. And when the child hears that voice and sees his or her mother for the very first time, it is something to behold.

I'll never forget the first time I noticed a mother on the stern deck, holding her little boy and pointing all around at the big, colourful world. 'That's the sky, and that colour is blue,' I could hear her telling him. 'And that is the ocean. Now you know how beautiful it is.'

It is said that the eyes are the windows of the soul.

Of the 60 million blind people in the world, 50 per cent could see with a twenty-minute ambulatory surgery much like the ones we did on this very first hospital ship port visit. In the years ahead, a Mercy Ship designed specifically to be a floating eye hospital will serve the entire Caribbean specialising in the wonderful medical field of giving back the gift of sight. Eye surgery and care is already a Mercy Ships cornerstone, and, in a way, I can't help but believe it has something to do with these first successes.

Here, in this small port on the edge of the Mexican coast, after ten long years, the Mercy Ship *Anastasis* finally fulfilled its destiny. It was now a hospital ship.

So now I got down to business. We began establishing relationships with governments. In the next few months, as we sailed the Mercy Ship around the Caribbean, we prepared our first protocol, a legal document we signed for our host governments, which described our potential and intent under their auspices. Our sailing year would centre around spending months at a time performing surgeries in needy ports upon invitation, then sailing back to European or US harbours for repairs, recruitment, and fund-raising in order to turn around, sail back, and perform surgeries for the world's poor once again.

In the next few months, while we solidified such full-time hospital ship plans and made Caribbean port visits and US maintenance stops, we also aided relief efforts in the wake of Hurricane Gilbert, and later, as we toured the US east coast, we docked with the *Good Samaritan* in Washington, DC, where we met as many US government officials as we could.

Finally it was time to go where Mercy Ships had been destined to go – since the first tactical plans developed in Switzerland a decade earlier – Africa. The way to get to Africa was via Europe.

On May 3, 1990, the Mercy Ship left New London, Connecticut, bound for Europe. It would be the first crossing of the Atlantic since our first 1982 voyage.

But strangely enough, this was the moment that Deyon and I decided to move off the ship, our family's home for a decade. And the decision would change the course of Mercy Ships in ways I could never have imagined.

LIFE BOAT

by John Dyson, excerpted from *Reader's Digest*, USA, June 2002

Dateline: Cotonou, Benin
6°21' N 2°23' E

A slim, rangy figure with short-cut hair and three gold bars on the shoulder tabs of his white shirt pauses on the gangway of the Anastasis. He gazes for a moment at the cluttered, chaotic, dilapidated port city, takes a deep breath and braces himself for the tough job ahead ... Dr Gary Parker goes ashore and drives to a nearby sports arena. Outside some 3,000 are standing, sitting, lying in the steamy equatorial heat. Waiting. For him. The maxillofacial surgeon may be their last hope ...

Angelle Koffi cooked meals to sell by the roadside. But her customers were few. People thought she was cursed, and they turned away from her. A tumour as large as a mango grew out of Angelle's cheek, distorting her nose and mouth sideways ... Shunned, the twenty-four-year-old orphan slept in an isolated hut. On the street, people ran at the sight of her ... only at church did she find some hope. One day, a visitor brought exciting news: 'The white ship is coming!'

Once in the stadium, Dr Gary Parker begins to look for good prospects for surgery. The UCLA-trained surgeon still has to turn away one in three who are too weak with advanced diseases to survive an operation ... Near the end of the day, a slim woman with a bowed head approaches him with a shawl covering her face. Parker tenderly folds back the cloth over Angelle's face. Her tumour is operable; he selects her for surgery.

'Welcome to Mercy Ship,' a nurse says to a hesitant Angelle, taking her hand. After a gruelling ten-hour surgery, she awakes fearful, her *face stiff and heavy. A nurse puts a mirror in her hand: There are bandages, stitches, and enormous swelling. But there is no tumour. All day she inspects her face. When Dr Parker comes to visit, she takes his hand in both of hers. 'I can give you nothing but my thanks,' she says through an interpreter, and her lopsided grin lights up the ship . . .*

One day, months later, a confident young woman walked gracefully down the gangway. In the pocket of her blue frock was a document that explained why the picture on her ID card no longer matched her face. When she got home, her pastor embraced her, whirling her round. 'Angelle, you are beautiful now!' he said. As Gary Parker was deftly sewing up an infant's cleft palate, a nurse told him about Angelle's welcome at home. 'That's why we're in business,' he said, smiling broadly. 'Angelle has got her life back.'

Ship's Log: 1989–1991

Garden Valley, Texas
$32^{0}21'$ N $95^{0}23'$ W

Lome, Togo
$6^{0}10'$ N $1^{0}21'$ E

Tema, Ghana
$5^{0}37'$ N $0^{0}1'$ W

CHAPTER 7
FINALLY TO AFRICA

We must use time wisely and forever realise that the time is always right to do right. – NELSON MANDELA

'You're moving where?'

If there was ever a bad time to move off the ship, this moment – on the eve of fulfilling Mercy Ships' floating hospital vision – would surely be it.

Yet that is exactly what happened. And no one was more surprised than I was. After living for ten years onboard the *Anastasis*, Deyon and I moved our four children off the ship. Why would we choose now, of all times, to move off the ship? The answer had to do with J. P., our handicapped son.

My life with Mercy Ships, I have noticed, has fallen into ten-year segments.

The first decade was spent living in an international city in the heart of Europe, letting the Mercy Ships vision form.

The next ten years were pioneering years for Mercy Ships, full of trials and errors.

The following decade I had always envisioned as time spent building Mercy Ships' infrastructure. That's exactly what happened, just not exactly as I'd planned or from where I planned it. And I was about to learn why. It would be the next in a series of lessons taught by my son.

How do we measure the value of a life? J. P. cannot speak, and yet just as Mother Teresa said so many years before, what we learned in caring, loving, and providing for him had translated into the Mercy Ships vision. J. P. continued to remind us each and every day of the value of the individual life and the God-given right to its quality. And once again, our son was telling us the way that Mercy Ships should go.

I just had to listen.

In 1989, John Paul, now thirteen, was very frustrated with life on the ship. Finally, the teachers at the onboard school came to us. They didn't say he was uneducable, but as politely as they could, they let us know something had to give. I remember looking at his special chair the teachers had brought into the kindergarten class where J. P. had gone every day for years, thinking how big it was in comparison to all the others, and I realised what was not being said. Being so big, he was no doubt more than a little frightening to some of the smaller children in the class.

To better care for J. P., it was time to move on.

The move was common sense, of course, and Deyon saw it clearly, but I took a little longer. I was involved in the ship at the deepest level of my soul. *How could I possibly leave the* Anastasis *at this point? This was my life. What would this mean for Mercy Ships?* Or that's what I was thinking, what I couldn't say out loud. Even the greatest ideas can flourish or falter on just such decisions. It took me quite a while to process it, but moving ashore turned out to be not only the right decision, but a pivotal one. Leaving the ship was exactly what I needed to do, not only for J. P., but for the future of Mercy Ships. I had been trying to grow the charity from onboard. And if I had stayed on the ship, Mercy Ships probably would have remained a small operation, limited in size and scope. And truthfully, I doubt if it would still be in existence today.

Where did we move? As strange as it may sound, we moved a ship-based charity to deep in the heart of landlocked Texas.

After our decision, I had gone ahead of the *Anastasis* to Europe in order to gain advice from old friends on where we should move to. I had a list for our move of things 'Required' on one side and things 'Desired' on the other side. And under 'Required', we had listed the most seemingly obvious need – a port location. We had outgrown our resource office facilities in Los Angeles, the most logical option. While we were considering all that, we were offered property in the Texas heartland – an eventual 400 acres in rural East Texas with an amazing amount of amenities for what we wanted to do. The only problem was that it happened to be hundreds of miles from the sea. So we set the idea aside and kept looking.

And that's when Henri André and his Swiss Atlantic experts once again entered the Mercy Ships story. 'If we can run a fleet of ships out of Switzerland, which will never have a port, you can do the same,' they said. All we truly needed was access to a good airport and telecommunications. So in September of 1989, we moved 'port location' from 'Required' to 'Desired', and ultimately, found ourselves saying yes to the spacious acreage with all its extras, hundreds of acres more than 600 miles from the gulf and almost 100 miles from the nearest international airport; the perfect place for a charity organisation focused on ships – perfectly improbable, that is. But that was exactly what we had come to expect from this Mercy Ships journey of ours.

In early fall 1989, we moved to the rolling hills of East Texas, and that has been our headquarters and our home ever since – a place where J. P. has the space he needs and deserves, and where Mercy Ships has the space to grow. We settled in and began to plot and plan the future.

The fact that we were sending the *Anastasis* back to Europe in preparation for Africa required deepened relationships with as many countries as possible. So, we studied our strategic plan once again and got to work developing legal and physical presences in seaport countries; rethinking the way we governed and managed work; and most important, forming an international board so that each of the nations where we opened support and resource offices would feel Mercy Ships was theirs as well as ours.

I had to let go and trust. What I have learned about authority is that the more you give away, the more you have. The more you try to keep, the more you lose. If the idea is the right one, then there's room for everyone. In other words, it was time to move from the bootstrap mentality, so important in the beginning, to the attitude that could take us to the next level – to a true global presence with potential as big as the sea itself.

I sensed a deep need to make myself more accountable. I had always had a legal board, but now that wasn't enough. If Mercy Ships was going to grow, I needed the wisdom and expertise of independent and knowledgeable individuals from all walks of life. We were already a floating global community of nations in so many ways, but to involve the rest of the world community meant thinking in new ways and persuading new thinkers to catch the Mercy Ships vision. We had the potential to encompass the best of all charity worlds – traditional, faith-based, humanitarian, corporate, and governmental – if we did this right. So I began to ask for help from some of the best minds in the world, captains of industry and medicine and commerce and diplomacy as well as captains of ocean-going ships – and I got it.

A group of these experts believed so deeply in Mercy Ships' global potential that they offered services far beyond my wildest hopes. Three men in particular worked closely with us, bringing the remarkable global expertise needed to fit our vision – William S. Kanaga, chairman of Arthur Young (now Ernst & Young) worldwide accounting firm, chairman of the US Chamber of Commerce, and chairman of the Centre for International Private Enterprise; William C. Turner, former ambassador to the Organisation for Economic Cooperation and Development (OECD); and Myron E. Ullman (Mike), a former White House Fellow, whose international business experience would soon extend around the globe – in Asia (the Wharf Holdings), the US (R. H. Macy & Co. and DFS Group, Ltd) and in Europe (LVMH Moët Hennessy Louis Vuitton).

They oversaw the structural, internal changes and provided the network of accountability needed to produce the future we all desired. Along with their unparalleled business acumen just when we needed it the most, they also brought hearts to serve the world's poor. The transformation they designed for Mercy Ships was amazing to watch.

Soon, we restructured into a legal multinational charity, beginning in Norway, Sweden, Denmark, Germany, Holland, Switzerland, and France. By the turn of the century, Mercy Ships would be a legal entity on five continents of the world. And all of it began when we moved ashore and began thinking like the global entity we wanted to be.

In the years to come, former British Prime Minister John Major would dedicate the International Support Centre, taking the long drive into the springtime Texas countryside to say memorable and warm words about our landlocked ship headquarters: 'It is from here in East Texas that medical and logistical supplies are organised and vessels dispatched. It is from here in East Texas that the healing flows.'

The move to Garden Valley, Texas, had been a risk. As usual, though, my friend Henri André had been right. By April 1990, with my family settling into life on solid ground and our organisational staff working from national offices around the world, the *Anastasis* set sail across the Atlantic towards Europe. I flew ahead to finish preparing the way.

The feel of history in the making seemed to be everywhere during that pre-Africa tour of Europe, one for the world history books, one for the Mercy Ships history books, and one for my own family history book. In June 1990, in the peaceful harbour of Kristiansand, Norway, as the Mercy Ship underwent maintenance, I felt the eyes of my Norwegian shipbuilding ancestors take a good look at this ship and this mountain-born descendant of theirs. Then, in July, we visited Poland.

The Berlin Wall had just come down, guards had abandoned Checkpoint Charlie, and Poland had its first free elections since World War II, beginning its historic transition from communism to a democratic society. And we wanted to do our small part to help. The *Anastasis* unloaded more than a million dollars of donations, including modern eye surgery equipment earmarked for the Gdansk hospital. Working double shifts, Solidarity longshoremen laboured with the ship's crew to unload the donations. And the Mercy Ship was in port on the day the shipyard workers brought down the huge bronze statue of 'Mother Russia' a few blocks away. Officials made speeches, and, in a fitting and memorable gesture, one man actually stepped forward and tweaked the statue's nose, to the crowd's applause.

In August, after a month in Rotterdam, the ship passed Lloyd's Register annual surveys.

We were good to go.

So we sailed to London, where we held medical receptions onboard, inviting health care professionals to visit the Mercy Ship in the hopes of recruiting their hands and their hearts to bring hope and healing to the poor.

One of the men who walked up the gangway was Sir John Chalstry. 'I am fascinated with what you do, and I believe in what you are doing and how you are doing it,' he said. 'I may soon have the opportunity to be the Lord Mayor of the city of London, and part of my charge will be to use the prestige of the office to help two charities of choice. My first choice will be St John's Ambulance. The second charity is not selected. I would like to suggest that you consider me making you the second charity. If you agree, we could use the Mansion House in London for a black-tie dinner to help make the charity known in the UK.'

I, of course, quickly agreed.

True to his word, Sir John Chalstry became Lord Mayor of London soon after, and we became his second 'charity of choice'. And just like that, we were propelled into the English public eye. The public awareness as well as the medical and financial partnerships that came from his support would fuel the next pivotal decade for Mercy Ships in ways we could never have imagined that night before we sailed to Africa.

While in Europe during that preparation time, over sixty-five thousand people visited the Mercy Ship. And as donations came in, we excitedly loaded the materials onboard for our first extended visit to Africa. We were ready for a whole new set of challenges – or we thought we were. As usual, no matter how much you think you are prepared, something unexpected always happens.

Our first stop was going to be Ghana. The plan was to stay several months. Our long-range goal was to spend longer and longer times each year serving both French and English-speaking Africa, all the way from Senegal in the north to Madagascar around the Cape. So, for this first big outing, we had chosen Ghana very deliberately to help our chances of success. We had all of our 'ducks in a row' strategically, for Ghana. The need had been assessed. It was an English-speaking country. It was economically stable. We even had former Mercy Ship staff who'd moved back there, which meant we had a local partner within the nation to help. We had met with the minister of health, we had been invited; all the right documents were signed and sealed, and we were ready, able, and willing to deliver.

But three weeks before departure, while docked in Denmark, we were in for a surprise.

I'll never forget the moment. We were in the middle of our government and civic reception in Copenhagen onboard the ship. I had just met the Ghanaian consul general when he leaned near and said, 'I need to speak with you.' I led him to my office and closed the door.

He told me that the head of state in Ghana had just contacted him and the decision to invite us had been 'frozen'.

I looked at him strangely. 'Frozen?'

'That is diplomatic parlance for "you can't come to Ghana",' he explained.

I couldn't find my voice for a few seconds. Finally, I said, 'Mr Consul General, we've put in two years of advance work. We have invested in surveys of health care needs; we are partnering with the ministry of health. We have it all organised, and we're only three weeks to departure. What do I do?'

His advice was to the point: First, go to another nation. Second, don't beg. 'If you come back to Ghana with your hat in hand, you will never get into any African nation,' he said. Then he added, 'There will be an answer.'

I don't know how long I sat there after the consul general left.

I should have been thinking about alternative plans, about how to explain this to donors and our new board and staff. And I especially should have been thinking about where to go from here considering I had no contacts in Africa other than in Ghana. But instead I was suddenly reminded that Mercy Ships did not belong to me. I remember that being the one clear thought, a reflection from out of nowhere, in the long minutes after the consul general dropped his bombshell.

And as I was thinking about Mercy Ships in that broad and sweeping way, a Swiss friend's name came to mind – Daniel Scherer.

Daniel once told me about his family, and I remembered that an uncle, a Dr DeLord, had been a famous French medical missionary in Togo years and years ago, building hospitals and clinics and teaching primary health care. So on an impulse, I picked up the phone and dialled Daniel and told him the situation, then mentioned that I remembered the story of his uncle.

He said, 'Don, it's interesting you should call and mention this, especially now. My uncle just returned from Togo.' The current head of state President Gnassingbe Eyadema had just flown him first class by Air France to Togo, and rolled out the red carpet – literally – to honour him for his medical service to the Togolese people so many years ago. While there, President Eyadema had asked him, 'Are there people like you in the world today who would do what you did for the people of Togo?'

'Well,' Daniel's uncle had said, 'my nephew knows a group.'

I didn't have time to think about how unusual that was at the time. I had a big problem to solve. So I levelled with Daniel: 'Would you mind asking your uncle to call the president back to see if he'd like that group to come – and come right now?'

Daniel agreed, and in no time, it seemed, he had phoned back to report that his uncle had phoned President Eyadema, explained that Ghana had frozen its invitation to the group he'd mentioned, so would Togo open the port for them to come instead?

President Eyadema's response? A resounding *yes!*

And so, the *Anastasis* sailed as planned three weeks from that day. But it sailed not to Ghana but to Togo.

Along the coast, tiny sea villages dotted the shoreline along the western edge of the African continent. It was a view that had barely changed in centuries. When we arrived in Lome, tugs swung the Mercy Ship portside to the dock, and we quickly arranged our first screening day, putting up announcements in clinics, churches, and government agencies, to help spread the word that a floating hospital was offering free medical services. All they had to do was come. And they did. We were quickly in business.

After operating only two or three weeks, some of our new friends came to warn us about what they had heard: 'The Ghanaian secret police are coming to the ship. They can't believe what you are doing.'

The port in Togo was only thirty minutes from the Ghana–Togo border, such as it is. Togo and Ghana are neighbouring nations. The French and the British had split the land along West Africa's Gold Coast during colonisation, dividing the land into two countries, but the boundary line doesn't exist for the Ewe people, one of the tribal affiliations of both populations. They move back and forth across the border as they've done for centuries, and so word travels back and forth with them. Obviously, Ghana's government officials had begun to hear about what we were doing. And now, it seemed, someone had sent their secret police to investigate. This did not sound good.

But yet again, we were in for a surprise.

'We made a mistake,' one of the police said. 'Would you cancel what you are doing in Togo and come to Ghana as you originally planned?'

We said no, that we had made a commitment and were going to stick to it. However, we did say that we would come to them next. And after our time in Togo ended in February, we sailed to Ghana and stayed for three months.

After a while, we discovered the reason Ghana froze our invitation. Rumours had reached each of the Ghanaian embassies in Europe that the Mercy Ship coming their way was really full of terrorists in surgeons' clothes, that we had AK-47s in our cargo holds and that when our gangway went down, like the Trojan Horse of Troy, enemy insurgents would rush into the country to stage a coup d'état. Of course, that panicked the nation of Ghana. They didn't know us. No one in Africa knew us yet.

That could have been the end of that story, but instead, we had a very important visitor near the end of our stay. We were only hours from sailing. All of a sudden, we heard a flurry of activity on the dock. Several military jeeps pulled up to our gangway. From one of them stepped the Ghanaian head of state, President Jerry Rawlings.

Our captain met him at the gangway, and I arrived immediately. He asked to see the ship, so I took him to the hospital where our surgeon, Dr Gary Parker, was finishing his examination of a cleft lip and palette patient. The boy was returning for one last postoperative follow-up. On the wall behind the boy, near where his father stood, were 'before' and 'after' snapshots of the little boy.

Studying the photos, President Rawlings asked the little boy, 'This was you?' The boy nodded happily. The president wanted to hear the whole story – what it was like to have surgery on the ship, how many other successful surgeries they'd seen, and on and on. Finally, after hearing all the father and son had to say, President Rawlings said to the captain, 'Would you assemble the remaining crew? I want to speak to them.'

The members of the crew assembled in the forward lounge. President Rawlings stepped to the microphone and said, 'I am here to apologise. I am the one who cancelled your invitation because I didn't believe people like you existed today. It was too good to be true. Now that I realise so many more of my countrymen could have been helped had I not made that decision, I feel I need to apologise to you.' He did not have to say that to us. The gesture spoke of the integrity of the man. His visit was a fitting and special end to a very strange beginning for Mercy Ships' Africa era.

On April 12, 1991, the big Mercy Ship turned and sailed back towards Europe, and that turn was also a literal turning point for us all. Togo and Ghana proved the floating hospital concept was the right one. The centre of the Mercy Ships' universe was now irrevocably its medical heart. This was our future, and West Africa's neediest countries would soon become the true home of the Mercy Ship *Anastasis*.

DOCUMENTARIES & ARTS: AFRICAN ER

Excerpt, BBC.co.uk for BBC-TV Documentary *Broadcast date: January 31, 2004*

Thousands of people have trekked hundreds of miles – sometimes from other countries – to the port of Freetown, Sierra Leone, just to find out if they are one of the lucky ones who will be picked to have their lives changed. This gathering of the country's outcasts is of biblical proportions. But it's not 'African Pop Idol'. People with terrible disfigurements, facial tumours the size of footballs, club feet, incontinence and blindness have turned up, desperate for surgery aboard a floating hospital . . .

Our presenter, Tash Monie, a glamorous south London girl who has never seen anything like this, watches as the volunteer nurses and doctors make the tough decisions about who should get treatment and who won't. It's an exhausting, heart-wrenching day. How do you decide who gets picked? And what does it feel like turning people away?

For Tash, the 'African ER' experience has just started. And it's going to be one hell of an experience. She plunges in at the deep end after she arrives in war-ravaged Sierra Leone – handing out water to the waiting crowds and hearing their desperate stories . . .

Ship's Log: 1991–2004

Puerto Cortes, Honduras
15°51' N 87°57' W

Abidjan, Ivory Coast
5°18' N 4°0' W

Suva, Fiji
18°8' S 178°26' E

Dakar, Senegal
14°40' N 17°22' W

Tamatave, Madagascar
18°9 S 49°25' E

CHAPTER 8
BRINGING HOPE AND HEALING

No one would remember the Good Samaritan if he only had good intentions. – MARGARET THATCHER

Of all the memories I have of those first hospital ship visits, the most vivid is the sight of people waiting in line during a screening day. Even now, after all these years, the sight is still incredibly moving. It is the moment we have been working towards for months. It is why we sail. Advance teams have gone ahead of the ship to advertise the medical screenings and the type of surgeries done onboard, hanging posters in health clinics and partnering with governmental, charitable, and religious organisations to spread the word.

People have come from all over the country, many travelling for days and sleeping overnight, hoping to secure a place near the front of the queue. As the word has spread through the years, the crowds have swelled to the point that government agencies have begun to open stadiums and sports arenas to hold the thousands who come and wait.

After the successful visits to Togo and Ghana, the Mercy Ship received invitations from more than a dozen nations. We have now sailed to places with names rarely heard in the developed world, places such as New Caledonia, Barahona, Lome, Conakry, Cotonou, Dakar, and Noumea. Needless to say, they are not tourist spots. They're not easily accessible, and are rarely in the headlines for any reason other than poverty and strife. Few of them are on our mental maps of the world, but each are forever on the heart maps of Mercy Ships crews.

Months of preparation were behind our first choice and we

quickly learned that it should always take that long. So, after that important first voyage, we tweaked our 'grid', a checklist to help our destination decisions go along with the official protocol I'd initiated after our first Mexico hospital ship operation. We had already decided we would only go to a country that invited us. So a written invitation from the country's government had to begin the process.

Next, we evaluated the depth of medical needs within the nation. We were committed to going to the very poorest of the poor – countries in the lowest one-third of the neediest nations in the world, as published by the United Nations Annual Human Development Index. Haiti is in the poorest tier, for instance, as are Sierra Leone and Liberia, which at the time of writing rank at the very bottom.

Next the technical questions must be answered. Is the harbour deep enough? Are there enough berths so we won't interfere with commercial shipping? Can they provide garbage disposal? Do they have enough fresh water to meet our need for one hundred tons a day? Will the port authorities waive fees?

After that comes a risk analysis. How stable is the country? How good is the port security? Is the nation on the verge of anarchy or revolution? We check with both the US State Department and the British Foreign Service for the latest information on any potential destination.

Then we meet with the minister of health and other health authorities to see if they will grant permission to the ship's medical staff to provide the surgeries, make visits to clinics, and undertake community health training. If permission is granted, then our various assessment teams – medical, dental, construction, water and sanitation, church and community health training – visit the port and surrounding villages.

When all of this is completed, the proposed port is presented to the Mercy Ships board and senior management, the final decision is made, we respond to the nation, and then put it on the schedule.

And all of that effort is to make this special day happen each year: the day we sail a Mercy Ship in to a country, lower the gangway, and step ashore to begin offering hope and healing however we can.

Of course, it's one thing for a government to trust you. It's another to be an ordinary citizen who has seen none of our official assurances. Africans had every right to be wary of ships docking at their ports with offers too good to be true. Not only were we battling the slave ship horrors of the past, we were also battling their spectres in the present. Each year, all along the sub-Saharan coastline, we hear rumours of a modern-day slave-labour ship that promises jobs and better lives to children, but that in reality offers forced labour and prostitution rings. Only word of mouth, straight from those helped and healed could truly build trust in Mercy Ships. And that is exactly what happened. Soon, people streamed into these port cities to wait in long lines for a chance to gain a surgical appointment card and the transformations those cards promised.

Medical screenings are a time when nearly the entire ship's crew gets involved by giving water, testing blood, checking temperatures, writing health histories, and escorting patients to the areas where doctors are examining people one by one. Most screening days can be as tragic as hopeful. Our Mercy Ships doctors have no choice but to turn away many patients we see because their diseases are too far advanced for us to help. All those who come are desperate and at their most vulnerable, and we strive to be worthy of their fragile trust. We have been so touched by some of the cases that we have set up a hospice branch to help support terminal cases during the months we are docked in port. The days ahead, the surgeries performed, and the life transformations they'll offer keep the team working, one by one, through the heart-rending crowd and down the long screening line.

A hospital ship lends itself to certain areas of expertise, and those are the ones we embraced – maxillofacial surgery, plastic surgery, orthopaedic surgery, eye surgery, and most recently, a specialty called vesico-vaginal fistula (VVF) repair for women. The stories that introduce each chapter of this book are examples of these specialties. The newborn Adam saved by the student Reginald was a cleft lip and palate surgery. Señora Camacho received a cataract surgery, and Mariama's son Ansu, whose pelvis was wounded by a rebel soldier's bullet, was an orthopaedic surgery. Edoh's need was for a maxillofacial surgery to remove her facial tumour.

All such stories have the power to break our hearts. But the power to change the endings of some is powerful medicine. Perhaps the best way to truly share the experience of a screening day is to tell one of these stories in depth.

Edoh's story is a perfect mirror for the drama of screening day for all concerned – and a great story. She came, literally tossed to us. What happened that day in Togo during the long screening day is a powerful story of mercy through the hands of gifted surgeons, but also the mercy extended by her crowd of fellow sufferers.

Her parents had all but given her up for dead when they heard about the hospital ship's return to their country. The tumour on the side of their daughter's face was the size of a grapefruit, and was slowly, relentlessly, closing off her airway. Her parents travelled 500 kilometres to bring her to the dock of Togo's port city, Lome. By the time they arrived with Edoh, the line was heartbreakingly long, and Edoh was gasping for breath. Her father, in desperation, lifted her above his head and someone beside him took her and passed her to the head of the line.

I have always been amazed at the inner calm of most Africans, even those in the direst distress. Our experience with screening day waiting lines is usually one of orderly quiet with hope in the air. That day the crowds were larger than we expected. In the five years since we last visited Togo, word had spread so far and wide that the city's officials and we were caught unprepared for the crush.

The long line that snaked back into the city had become a massive crowd. And as the crowd was pressing dangerously up against the dock's fencing where we had directed the line around for the screening tests, we were forced to close the iron gates momentarily for crowd control. But then one of our security crew saw a child with a grotesque facial tumour being passed towards the front, above the crowd, person to person, hand to hand, and could hear her desperate gasps for breath.

Everyone in that line was suffering beyond anything most people in the Western world can fathom and yet these people instantly saw a child in an even more desperate, immediate need of help. And as the crowd continued to be pushed against the fence between the screening area and the line, one by one those hands moved little Edoh to the front and then over the fence into the waiting arms of John Syrbe, a Mercy Ships crew member.

What made this even more poignant was that John had been born with a cleft lip and palate, endured nine operations in his young life, and had recently undergone further corrective surgery onboard. John took one look at Edoh, heard her gasps, and rushed her to the surgeons who performed a tracheotomy. In the months ahead, Edoh underwent a series of operations, including one in Germany, to correct the damage done by the tumour. Then one day, right before we sailed, she went home with her parents to grow up like any other normal African child.

Edoh's medical problem is not uncommon in West Africa. Mercy Ships has performed many of these operations to remove jaw tumours, saving countless people from suffocation, starvation, and death. But such deformities often hold more suffering than just potential death. If you have a physical deformity, not only do you have little hope for the future, but you are usually an outcast. In some remote villages, midwives still snatch newborn babies with cleft lip and palates and bury them alive. In others, the family shuns mother and baby because they believe the devil has touched them both.

Many people in the developing world live daily with the fear of a curse being put on them. And such deformities are, more often than not, seen as the result of such curses. Those who have such a condition have little hope. They can't be educated, few people will employ them, and people often run from or even throw stones at them. They are left to a life of begging or, worse, a life lived in the shadows of the only civilisation they've ever known – a non-person, hiding in the bush, shunned, literally waiting to die.

We've learned to leave time for a second screening, because only after news of dramatic success stories filter back into the villages do many with the worst disfigurements have the courage to come out of hiding. The doctors who volunteer from around the world are often surprised when patients wince or shrink away as they reach to examine them. The patients do not draw back from fear of physical pain, but because that moment is often the first time in years another human has dared to touch them.

After the screening schedule has been filled, in the coming weeks people just like Edoh will fill the beds of the ship's recovery wards. Most of their faces will be swollen, bruised, and bandaged, but without fail, on the first early-morning rounds the next day, most of them will borrow mirrors to admire themselves. When they see the medical staff, they turn their heads and flex their new smiles. I'll never forget the first time I saw a mother holding her little boy who could now see again, standing at the ship's stern, showing him the world. It was the same amazing moment as I'd been privileged to witness in Mexico, but now it was happening on the other side of the world.

And as the wards fill up during the months we're in port, we get to know these people very well, and often become very close to them.

But it's not that way when we first meet them on screening day. The hope and pain in the eyes of most of those in line is nearly always mingled with a touch of fear.

'What do we have to do?' is a constant question.

'Nothing,' we say. 'There is no catch. Everything is free. We treat everyone without regard to race, religion, sex, or creed.'

This is delicate territory. We are serving the most vulnerable of the vulnerable. Who wouldn't do or say anything to be healed of one's horrible suffering? And who wouldn't find it hard to believe such a gift comes without one string attached? But that's the beauty of Mercy Ships. Offering the gift of health in any context but sheer altruism and love has deep flaws. And so we go out of our way to be sensitive to the fears of those we screen, those people hoping against all hope to be able to receive such a gift.

Within days, though, everything has changed. The relationships we form with those who come onto a ship for medical help almost defy description. Let me try to describe it in another context. When you meet someone for the first time, there is a relationship timeline. You don't expect them to be considered a close, intimate family friend within the first several meetings. In some cultures that requires twenty years, so a person can have only so many of such deeply bonded relationships in a lifetime. And if you are an outsider who doesn't speak another person's language, who is not from the other person's culture, your attempts to have a close relationship with that person might take a lifetime to form, if it happens at all.

But when you sail into a port city and you perform a life-changing surgery on a family member, all of that evaporates. Twenty years collapses into twenty-four hours. And all of a sudden, you are no longer an outsider. Instant bonding takes place. Barriers are down. So the Mercy Ships crew must tread very softly in the beginning, if we are truly doing what we say we are: putting love into action and offering medical care with no strings attached.

As time goes by we often find ourselves having to explain the Mercy Ships way of life. We are a hospital ship charity committed to bringing hope and healing to the world's poorest of the poor, we say. Some are here because of their faith, putting it into everyday action, some are here because of their expertise, giving of their talents and gaining experience they could never find anywhere else in the civilised world. Some are here because they love the sea, and they want to experience a seafaring way that is not all about the bottom line – something worthy – wanting to make a lasting difference in the world.

'You mean you don't get paid to do this?' our patients often ask.

'No. We do it because of a deeper purpose,' is my usual answer.

And actually, I think we aren't that unusual. I'm convinced that the desire for deeper purpose resides within everyone. It's built-in. We truly do want to help our neighbour if we have the chance. I've observed this dynamic in the inner cities of not only the United States but nations around the world, as well as the faraway places of sub-Saharan Africa, the Middle East, the South Pacific, and Asia – people doing a little-bit for the next person, trying to make the world a better place, even if it's only in the tiniest of ways. The fellow sufferers who helped Edoh by lifting her over their heads despite their own pain are perhaps the best example of this impulse in us all.

A recent trends analyst described Mercy Ships as a non-traditional charity creating modern partnerships with individuals, corporations, churches, charities, and governments. Humans make up organisations, and the vast majority of humanity has this built-in desire to leave the world a better place – somehow, someway – if given the chance.

Interestingly enough, a funny thing happens when the built-in desire becomes action. For those poorest of the poor whose lives come in contact with a Mercy Ship, they never forget the day everything changed with the help of a surgeon's scalpel and hundreds of pairs of loving, ship-worthy hands. But it goes both ways. When you reach out to serve the poor, you discover it is they who give to you, not just the other way around. Their grace, patience, and gratitude in response to the smallest act of kindness changes those privileged to serve them.

Actions speak loudest on a Mercy Ship. A respect for others, wherever they are, whatever their culture, is a guiding tenet of a every port visit, during screening day and throughout each individual's stay onboard. Armed with that respect and governmental invitations, all that is truly necessary for us to gain trust is a few testimonials from transformed relatives, friends, and neighbours dancing back down the ship's gangway.

And that's exactly what has happened.

THE STORY OF VVF WOMEN

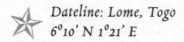 *Dateline: Lome, Togo*
6°10' N 1°21' E

Akou had already given birth to children, but when another came along in 1996, she could not deliver him. For four days she laboured and finally, with her son born dead, she no longer had control of her bladder. Her husband left her. She tried to make a living by selling goats, but people didn't like to come near her because of her smell. Her husband's other three wives shunned her, often laughing at her, pointing their fingers and making fun of her always wet skirts. They believed she would die.

Millions of women live daily with the same humiliation and dejection. Often barren and with a stench that drives them to seclusion, they stay in the shadows with no voice to speak out against their unjust suffering.

They suffer with vesico-vaginal fistulas (VVFs) and experts estimate they number in the millions worldwide. When obstructed labour causes a fistula or hole to form between the bladder and vagina, women find the constant trickle of urine, and sometimes faeces, makes normal life impossible. Women who have undergone VVF surgeries onboard a Mercy Ship also reveal other causes: rape at a young age, accidents, or the slip of a knife while having a Caesarean delivery.

In a part of the world where a woman's worth lies in her ability to bear children and usefulness as a wife, these women are often abandoned. And so they suffer alone. Akou, too, thought she would die from her misery. But she didn't, and finally, after seven years of suffering, she danced down the gangway of the Mercy Ship, dry after her own successful surgery onboard.

SHIP'S LOG: 1990–2000

Cotonou, Benin
6°21' N 2°23' E

Banjul, The Gambia
13°27' N 16°35' W

Conakry, Guinea
9°30' N 13°43' W

CHAPTER 9
HEART OF AFRICA

The true neighbour will risk his position, his prestige, and even his life for the welfare of others. – MARTIN LUTHER KING, JR

'Don, I have a delegation down here from the United States. They would like to tour the ship,' the gangway watchman informed me. 'What should I do? The ship is closed on Sunday.'

'Open the ship,' I said. 'I'll come down immediately.'

Deyon and I had come to Togo with the board members. Once a year, our International Board's executive committee members travel to one of our ships to observe the life and work of a Mercy Ship in action. We had already been there five days, and we were leaving the next day. Most of the board members were visiting the city, but Deyon and I had chosen to stay onboard and rest. About 3 p.m. in the afternoon, the US delegation appeared at the bottom of our gangway.

The group was in Togo as part of a multinational group monitoring the Togo presidential elections, and while there had heard about a Mercy Ship docked in the port. They'd like to know more, they had told the crew member on watch.

So, Deyon and I gave them a tour.

The group included the Togolese ambassador to the United States Akoussoulelou Bodjona, US Congresswoman Corrine Brown, and Martin Luther King III. Congresswoman Brown, upon her return to the States, introduced Mercy Ships to the black caucus of the US House of Representatives for endorsement and support for what we are doing in Africa – a wonderful gesture. Martin Luther King, president of the Southern Christian Leadership Council, was representing the SCLC as an official delegate observer of the election process.

It was an honour to meet them all. Meeting Martin Luther King Jr's son was not only a surprise, but an unusually significant moment for me. I have no idea what his thoughts were; if he knew he was embodying all the symbolism of his father's civil rights history, especially standing as we were on a ship docked along what once was Africa's slave coast. But as they left, I felt the weight of history surrounding me.

To work with the African continent is to be engaged with history almost every moment of the day. You can't help but face the past even as you work to heal old wounds as only hospital ships can.

As mentioned earlier, the rumours of slave ships were still very much alive along this coast, hundreds of years after slavery was abolished. They had grown to the point that in 2001, news spread around the world concerning a suspicious freighter believed to be just such a slave ship, carrying children away to forced labour or worse. A ship named the *M/V Etireno* had become a 'rogue' ship, having been turned away from Cameroon and Gabon, and was now being turned away from Benin as well. The rusting ship had docked within sight of the *Anastasis* there in Benin, before it was forced back to sea. News photographers and reporters touring the *Anastasis* during that week found themselves asking permission to shoot footage of the *Etireno* from our ship's top deck to feed to their home offices.

Child labour is common in parts of Africa, and child trafficking has long been known as an African problem. During that time, the United Nations estimated that more than two hundred thousand children were working as slave labourers. The charges were never confirmed about the rogue ship, even though officials feared there was truth to the rumours, but global media including CBS, BBC, CNN, and major international newspapers carried stories of the suspicion around the world and back. That's how this dreaded chapter of the past lives on in this part of the world.

In 1999, Benin's President Kérékou became the first African leader to publicly apologise for African involvement in the slave trade, and soon afterwards, Ghanaian President Jerry Rawlings offered an apology as well. Kérékou held a historic reconciliation conference to bring together the descendants of all those involved – from representatives of the historic slave cities to heads of state to descendants of slaves.

In 2000, the *Anastasis* visited The Gambia, the African country where Alex Haley's famous ancestor lived. I was one of the millions of people deeply affected by the literary phenomenon *Roots*, Alex Haley's chronicle of the tracing of his 'roots' back through family legends to the African ancestor sold into slavery from the Gambia River. And the impact of that book was not only felt in the West. Africans are equally aware of the saga, especially Gambians.

George Haley, Alex Haley's brother, was the US ambassador to his ancestral country in 2000, and we were privileged to meet him. Inside the ambassador's residence hung a huge mural of the Haley family tree, tracing those famous roots all the way back to the Gambian who was forced into slavery and sent by slave ship to America.

Ambassador Haley invited several of us to take a trip up the Gambia River in the US Embassy's small boat, to villages we wanted to visit inland. As we motored up the Gambia River, I could almost see the years recede. After only a few miles inland, the country looked as it must have looked two hundred years ago. Ambassador Haley, Dr Gary Parker, and I discussed a lot of things on that trip, but one comment Ambassador Haley made deeply affected me in that special setting. As terrible as slavery was, I recall him saying, he couldn't help but wonder where he might be had his famous ancestor Kunte Kinte not been taken as a slave. Wasn't it amazing that a 'seventh generation son of a slave could come back to serve as ambassador to his ancestor's homeland'?

The *Anastasis*' executive director Daslin Small, a Jamaican-born, Toronto-educated woman of African descent, has expressed the same full-circle feelings. The first time she sailed to Africa on a ship, she said her 'heart choked up'. Onboard with her were more than forty West Africans, along with hundreds of Europeans, Britons, and Americans. 'Here I was,' she said, 'the descendant of Africans sold onto slave ships leading a crew of descendants of both slaves and slavers on a ship of healing back to Africa.'

During that trip down the Gambia River with Ambassador Haley, we met the village elders of Brikama, who wanted to know about our hospital ship, about the surgeries and the community development projects we'd begun to do on land. It was the first time Mercy Ships had been to The Gambia. They didn't know us, and we didn't know them. I did know, however, that the city elders were Muslim. I also knew many of the parents had been afraid to bring their children to the medical screenings near the hospital ship because of the modern-day slave ship rumours. I could only imagine what they were thinking.

What do they want to hear? I wondered. *What is the most important thing I could say to them?*

In this land where history is mostly passed on by word of mouth, I knew these leaders could tell me which tribes were raided and which tribes participated with the Europeans in the slave raids centuries ago. So, with the help of Dr Schneider who spoke the local language Mandinka fluently, I decided to talk about our common history: 'Ships have many purposes in history, some good and some bad. You know that ships have come to this river before, and your people have been abused. But I represent ships that are totally different. They are not slave ships but ships of hope. Not ships of aggression and abuse, but ships that bring healing. We are here wanting to partner with you. We want long-term relationships based on mutual trust.'

At the end of our presentation, the Muslim tribal chieftains asked, 'Could we pray together before we finish this meeting?'

Taken aback, I quickly agreed.

They said, 'Here is how we want to do it, to recognise our mutuality and trust. We want to pray for your ship. We want to ask God to bless your ship. We will pray in our way as Muslims. And you pray in your way as followers of Jesus.'

And so we did.

After months of work in The Gambia, we received a letter from President A. J. Yahya Jammeh. 'We cannot thank you enough,' he wrote. 'Not only have you treated my people and taken care of them, but you have also taught them valuable lessons, the most important being love and respect.' But he also put those beautiful words into action by personally underwriting the costs of two of his countrymen to serve onboard our hospital ship.

The Muslim village elders and their prayer brought home another reality of Africa. To work in Africa is to live not only with the results of history, but also with history in the making – the politics of our time. And that includes the Muslim/Christian tensions that face us in the 21st century.

Many people don't think of African nations as being Muslim. But West Africa, sub-Saharan Africa, is a land of Muslim countries. Many are 50 to 90 per cent Muslim. Several, such as Guinea, are almost 100 per cent Muslim. And Africa hasn't escaped the same inbred tensions between their own Christian and Muslim factions, equally as bloody and explosive as the rest of the world's, and growing alarmingly more so each year. Other countries, far from the Middle East, countries we hope one day to visit with a Mercy Ship, are also Muslim by faith. Indonesia, for instance, is the largest

Muslim nation in the world. And that makes the questions concerning our motives even more loaded from a geopolitical point of view.

You can imagine, then, how sensitive and doubly cautious the Mercy Ships crew has to be in a Muslim nation when our motives are questioned. 'What do we have to do to be helped by your surgeons?' they ask, waiting for the hook.

'Nothing,' we reply, as always. 'We do it for free. There is no catch.' In a Muslim context, though, the question then takes on another dimension: 'Is there a religious creed I have to subscribe to?'

'Absolutely not,' we answer, as we always answer. 'We will perform the surgery on you or your child without any prequalifications whatsoever, and we will send you home.'

Then we explain that there has never been any pressure or coercion on an individual as a precondition to receiving our services or help of any kind, and that there never will be. Before we enter any nation, we sign a protocol with top government officials to assuage such fears. We have been invited back to every nation where a Mercy Ship has served, including Muslim nations.

Interestingly enough, I initially declined the very first invitation we received from a Muslim nation. The nation was Guinea, which is almost 100 per cent Muslim. The invitation came during our first trip to Togo. I decided not to accept it. And soon I received a visit from a handful of the nation's civic leaders and health authorities who were in Togo for a World Bank meeting.

'What might we say to persuade you to bring your hospital ship to our people?' they asked.

I had a list of reservations, I told them, trying to be as polite as I could.

'Would you mind sharing them?' one of them asked.

'First,' I explained, 'I don't think we are ready.' We had just experienced our very first year in Africa. At the time they visited us, we had eighteen different nationalities in the medical department alone – doctors, dentists, nurses, and lab technicians from Africa, Europe, Australia, New Zealand, the Dominican Republic, and the United States. And while we were learning quickly how to adapt and work with each other's many different cultures and languages, I truly didn't think we were ready to work in a Muslim nation – yet.

'Second,' I admitted, 'I'm not certain we could get the assurances needed that we won't be the targets of the radical Islamic elements within a Muslim nation.' Even then it was a threat worldwide.

On I went, going down my list, one by one. One by one, they countered every concern. Still, I was very hesitant, and told them so.

Then one of them said perhaps the one thing I could not ignore: 'Do you know of the hospital ship *Hope*?'

'Yes,' I said. 'It's one of the models we studied to become what we are.'

'Did you know the *Hope* visited here twenty-five years ago?'

That got my attention.

'And did you know,' he added, 'that our nation's families still talk about the wonderful work the ship did here, to this day?'

As you might imagine, we went to Guinea. In fact, we went the very next year. That encounter taught me a valuable lesson about the common ground of medicine, its incredible power, and the hope it offers as a basis on which mutual trust can grow.

And I also learned that with much of the Muslim world, surprisingly enough, the way to engage their culture with respect often means meeting them on common ground.

Two of my favourite Mercy Ships stories involve Muslim patients, offering hope beyond religion and politics through the mercy of medicine.

The first one begins with the crafting of artificial eyeballs. During our visit to Guinea, a Muslim judge, unable to find help for his little boy, came to our screening day.

'Do I have to become a Christian first? Pray in Jesus' name and follow him?' the judge had asked, warily, during the screening.

We told him we would operate on his little boy the same as we would anyone else, with no preconditions whatsoever.

'But you are Christian,' he said, studying our reactions carefully.

'Most of us are but not all of us,' we told him. 'What we do is an expression of God's love, much like Mother Teresa has done in Calcutta. The model for our efforts is the example of Jesus. And for Mercy Ships that includes healing those who are sick, with no strings attached.'

He considered that for a moment, and then allowed our team to examine his little boy. Glaucoma was destroying the little boy's eye. When the doctors said they could provide a glass eye, the judge allowed them to take his son onboard. The boy, whose name was Alseny, stayed onboard for ten days, time enough for the surgery, healing, and fitting of the prosthetic eye. His father and older brother came to see him every day.

Prosthetist Paul Moehring, a dental technician from Texas who joined the crew to make dental bridges and crowns, had quickly become the creative genius behind such custom needs as artificial teeth, ears, eyes, noses, even prostheses models for jaw replacement operations. We gave him a closet-size office crammed under the bow of the ship where he stuffed his gizmos along with a stereo that wafted Mozart down the corridors as he worked.

I was there when he made three prosthetic eyes for Alseny. After he made one to fit Alseny's eight-year-old face, Paul then measured the diametre of his father's and older brother's eyes, in order to estimate the size of two larger eyeballs – one to fit Alseny in his early to late teens, and a third one to fit him as an adult.

When little Alseny saw his face in a mirror for the first time with his new artificial eye, his smile was so bright, it almost lit up the entire room. And soon, he was holding the box with the other eyeballs ready for his future face as well.

On the day that the judge, along with his elder son, came to take the boy home, some of the civic and government leaders who had opened the door for us to come to Guinea happened to be onboard visiting us. We were all standing in the reception area when little Alseny, beaming, came rushing into the room and ran to his older brother, who had not yet seen his new eye. The brother twirled him around, both of them laughing excitedly at his new 'look'.

The judge turned to me in front of the Guinea leaders and said: 'This is my youngest boy, and I love him greatly. Other children threw stones at him and called him names, yelling that "the Great Satan" had entered him. I couldn't find any help nor could I protect him, even though I am a judge in my nation's second largest city. Then I came to you on this hospital ship and you helped us for free.'

He smiled, watching little Alseny show his brother his box of eyeballs. 'Muslims are told in the Koran that the good Muslim is to read the Injil – what you call the Gospels – and to honour the People of the Book, all Jews and Christians,' he continued. 'I have not become a Christian, but because you have helped my son when no one else could, I am reading the Injil to learn more about this loving side of Allah, and . . . ' he added, with a wink, 'I'm praying in Jesus' name, just in case.'

A second story involves another such surprise, with a twist. An ophthalmologist from Texas, a Jewish Christian proud of his heritage, has volunteered on our ships several times. On this trip, his very first patient was a blind African mullah, the religious leader of a mosque. The mullah told the doctor through a translator, 'I want you to operate on my eyes so I can once again study the Koran and teach my people how to live.'

When the doctor heard this, he excused himself from the operating room to go outside. His internal dialogue went something like this: *I've just taken two long flights to the other side of the world. I miss my wife and kids. I'm losing thousands of dollars in operating revenue in my home practice, and my first patient is a Muslim mullah? Is this really what I should do?*

And after a few tense moments, he had the impression that he should do the best possible surgery he could because God loved the mullah as much as God loved him. So he returned to the operating room. What he didn't know was that the nurses had been talking to the mullah, and had mentioned that the doctor was Jewish. Guess who had the problem now?

The mullah, all too aware of what was happening in the Middle East, suddenly wasn't so sure he wanted this Jewish doctor, with his set of surgical knives, working on him.

Here was the geopolitical situation of the world in a microcosm, and it was happening onboard our ship, right before our very eyes. Finally, the mullah consented and the doctor performed the surgery. All went well.

Before the doctor left to go home, one of our follow-up team returned to the ship looking for him. 'We want you to know what is happening, before you leave,' the team member explained. The mullah told them that although he was skilled in knowledge of the Koran, he had never experienced such a loving community. He remembered our explanation of the mercy found on Mercy Ships. Since we were People of the Book, and studying our book was part of a good Muslim's duty, he had told the people in his mosque that the only way to discover this loving nature of the character of God would be through studying the Injil. So, the mullah procured video equipment and was playing a video version of the gospel of Luke in his mosque to teach them what he learned from a Jewish doctor about a God of love.

Sometimes we find ourselves working with the all too recent wounds of war, the kind of history humanity knows all too well. Mercy Ships doctors have performed war-related surgeries after civil wars in such places as Sierra Leone and Nicaragua – maimings from machete attacks, limb losses from land mines, all the things you imagine during war's atrocities. Often, the walking wounded come to us through the country's medical, religious, and humanitarian agencies, sometimes brought by one of these selfless workers personally. The story of Tamba is a marvellous example.

When rebel forces swept through his village, Tamba told us that he remembered hearing gunfire and screaming. He immediately joined a stampede of villagers running for their lives. They all ran for a low bridge between the village and the bush to hide, but the rebels followed. Tamba jumped from the low bridge and took cover. When he felt a prod by a soldier's boot, he knew it was over. He caught the sudden movement of a machete slicing through the air toward his neck. He ducked sideways and the next thing he knew he was clutching a pulpy mass that had been the right side of his face. He heard the soldiers laughing as they left him to die. 'You're good for nothing now, friend,' one of the soldiers had sneered.

Somehow Tamba stumbled through the bush until an older couple found him and took him in. The days and weeks blurred as infection set in on what was left of his face. He finally decided to try to return home to die. While there, he met a human rights worker named Eva who took Tamba to a nongovernmental organisation, Médecins Sans Frontieres (Doctors Without Borders), where their medical personnel began to treat him. When they'd done their best, he was still missing a large part of his cheeks, one side of his nose, and most of the flesh covering both his upper and lower jaws.

Tamba returned to his job as an auto mechanic and learned to get through his village by keeping his head down and his face covered. But each glimpse in a mirror pushed him further into depression. One day, Eva told him of a Mercy Ship coming to Freetown. Tamba shrugged. He wasn't interested. He'd lost all hope long ago. Finally, friends from MSF persuaded him to go with them to the ship's screening. There, the doctor he met uttered words he never thought he'd hear. '*I think we can help you.*'

Three surgeries would be required, but soon he'd have a face again. After his first surgery, the nurses began to notice that his eyes were twinkling above the bandages. One day, he joked about the day he'd have to shave the moustache that would now grow from the parts of his scalp the doctors had used to rebuild his face. Finally the day came when he was able to look himself in the mirror and smile once again.

Injuries from traditions may break our hearts most of all, because they are so preventable. We see our share of botched procedures. The African tradition of female genital mutilation known as FGM has attracted worldwide outrage in recent years. Millions of girls are subjected to female genital mutilation every year. The story that tugs at my heart is little Kumbuna. Two and a half years old, chestnut eyes, tiny braids around her head like a halo, babbling in a Serahule dialect, she was cheerful and healthy except for one thing – a botched female circumcision that made urinating all but impossible for the toddler.

Ignoring the protest of a father who demanded that his daughter remain untouched, Kumbuna's grandmother, a powerful figure in their tribe, insisted the ritual take place. But the tradition was shoddily done and the razor cuts resulted in scar tissue forming over her urethra. Her mother brought her to a Mercy Ship where the doctors performed the surgery she needed. The team knew little Kumbuna's healing was going to be incredibly painful. So they kept Kumbuna and her mother in the ship's ward, so she could be given medicine to help her through the awful pain.

'The grandmother is now dead,' her mother told the nurses. 'If not, I would bring her here so she could see what she has done.' Weeks later, both mother and child returned for her final post-operative check. They were both smiling. They were both happy. The scars will always be with Kumbuna but the pain is gone. And we can only hope that her future will be one that will see an end to this barbaric female ritual.

As we began to see such specific problems facing so many African women, Mercy Ships vowed to bring justice as well as healing to them. In recent years, we've made vesico-vaginal fistula (VVF) surgeries one of our specialties. A 2004 BBC Worldwide report highlighted the work of Mercy Ships in battling the problem. The report called it a 'female medical crisis the world is only just beginning to understand'.

Childbearing in the developing world can be life-threatening, with the mother in as much danger as the child. But the mother – like Akou, whose story opened this chapter – is also in danger of damage done to other organs, including the bladder that can cause non-stop urine leakage. That leads to embarrassment and ostracisation for the vast majority of African women. They face the same potential social problems as those with other serious disfigurements – abandonment by their husbands and families, and sometimes even their children are taken away from them. So Mercy Ships has begun to offer special surgeries to correct this condition and restore women to wholeness.

Ethiopia's Addis Ababa Fistula Hospital, world-renowned for its pioneering work in fistula surgeries, trains and sends surgeons all over the developing world to help organizations like ours. The hospital was founded by Australian doctors Catherine and Reg Hamlin in 1975, and has successfully operated on more than twenty thousand women.

After her husband's death, Catherine continued the work and ultimately was nominated for the 1999 Nobel Peace Prize, immortalising their story in the book *The Hospital by the River*. Two of their specialists came to offer their services during our Sierra Leone visit in 2003, the current director Dr Andrew Browning and a special woman named Mamitu Gafhi who has performed more than two thousand surgeries, and whose own story is remarkable.

As a young Ethiopian bride, Gafhi endured six days of excruciating labour. Her baby was stillborn and complications left her with VVF. After a series of surgeries and more complications, she was told the hard truth – her condition was too extreme for correction. She would never be healed. Mamitu turned the tables and dedicated her life to helping other women with VVF who could be healed. She stayed on at the Ethiopian hospital, learning to perform VVF procedures on her own. Along with both Drs Hamlin, Mamitu Gafhi was cited on the Gold Medal for Surgery from the Royal College of Surgeons in London. Forty years later, she is still performing the surgery. Only four doctors worldwide have performed more VVF surgeries than this one African woman who decided not to give up by giving back.

Every woman after VVF surgery onboard a Mercy Ship is given a new dress as a symbol of her brighter future. And quite often, a group of these women will burst into joyous dance and song after their recovery, dancing down our gangways into normal life. It is a sight to behold. And you can imagine how the crew loves joining each and every celebration.

To interact with Africa is to work with the past and the present, in all its forms and challenges. With the weight of history and politics always near, these amazing years in Africa have taught us so much. We aim to act as healing agents in every possible way; we meet nations where they want to be met, through dialogue and relationship building, focusing on what we have in common.

In this way, sailing with mutual respect and care, Mercy Ships should continue to enjoy the humbling privilege of offering hope and healing in every port of call. And when I doubt this is true, I hear the Guinea Muslim leaders: 'Did you know our families still talk about the time the hospital ship *Hope* visited here twenty-five years ago?'

My hope is that years from now the same will be said for the hospital fleet called Mercy Ships, that they become a part of history, too – a tool of reconciliation for all.

FROM THE BRIDGE

Excerpted from *Mercy Ships News*, all editions, March 2000

 Bulletin:
Latest News of Mercy Ships Fleet

Caribbean Mercy

The ship's cargo holds were full as she left in February for her return medical port call to El Salvador. Telemundo, a Latin television station, has agreed to cover the President and First Lady's visit to the ship . . .

Anastasis

While sailing from Cape Town to The Gambia, the crew sterilised the OR suite. On February 1, following two successful surgical screening days during which 386 patients received appointments, surgeries got underway.

In the town of Brikama, about an hour's drive from Banjul's harbour, the dental team established their dental clinic. On Feb. 3–4 the village medical team began their daily clinics in the Kombo Central District at Kassa Kunda, an area which does not have easy access to medical facilities . . .

New Ship (soon to be Africa Mercy)

Architectural plans have been drawn up to convert the ship to a hospital vessel and work on the vessel continues at a steady pace. The new crew is setting up operations onboard.

The Naming Ceremony for the new ship has been set for April 4th. People from all over the world are flying to Newcastle for this milestone event . . .

Ship's Log: 1990 to Present

Longitude/Latitude: The World

CHAPTER 10

To the Ends of the Earth

If there are poor on the moon, we will go there too. – MOTHER TERESA

It takes nearly 30,000 miles to circumnavigate the globe by ocean. By the turn of the century, the *Anastasis* had sailed 182,831 miles. The combined miles of all Mercy Ships as we sailed into the 21st century was easily the equivalent of a dozen trips around the world – and counting.

After that pivotal winter of 1991, we found a routine, sailing along the West African coast and back again to Europe. Except for one year when the ship returned to the United States, and another when it went to South Africa, the *Anastasis* has plied that same route to this day spending four to seven months at one or two countries a year before sailing back to Europe for maintenance, recruiting, and fund-raising. Each year, our screenings became larger, the medical volunteers busier, the recovery wards fuller, and the partnering opportunities on land more plentiful. The next year, in 1992, our two ports of call were the Ivory Coast and Guinea.

The third year, Sierra Leone was our only port, but not actually by choice. You can't live and work on a ship and not have your share of nautical misadventures. That year, while in Sierra Leone, the ship's boiler broke down. Taking a positive approach, the crew made the most of it by extending the outreach to that country until a brand new boiler could be installed. After that, we sailed to the US for the required maintenance, recruiting, and fund-raising routine. Then in 1994–95 we returned to Africa for a long visit to Ghana.

In 1996, after a return visit to Togo, we sailed due south. Apartheid had just been abolished. So in the same spirit as our visit to Poland in 1990, we sailed to South Africa to support that amazing freedom event. The South Africa visit was the only time in which the *Anastasis* could 'do it all' in one country – dry dock maintenance, recruitment, and fund-raising, as well as medical and dental treatments. That allowed us to spend over an entire year on the continent of Africa. Ahead were visits to Benin, Guinea, The Gambia, and Senegal. Then came the long-awaited return to Sierra Leone.

When Mercy Ships first visited Sierra Leone in 1992–93, some of the patients who underwent surgeries needed follow-up operations. So we had promised to return in the next year or so. We gave these patients 'return appointment cards' for the follow-up care. Little did we know that we would not be able to return to Sierra Leone for a decade. Civil war erupted almost immediately after we left the country. When we did return in 2001, the crew didn't know who would, or even could, return after the long rebel war.

When I think of that return visit, and the anticipation the crew felt waiting to see if any of their former patients would arrive, I think of Patrick Coker. Before his surgery, Patrick lived with a jaw tumour that had been growing since he was eight years old. In 1993, chief medical officer Dr Gary Parker performed two operations on Patrick, removing the tumour and affected portions of his lower jaw, and inserting a titanium implant. Patrick spent two weeks in the recovery ward as he healed. His next surgery would replace the titanium plate with one of his own bones. When the ship sailed, Patrick had his return card in hand for that follow-up operation.

Then the civil war began. During those years, Patrick married and had three children. Anticipating the horrific rebel attack on

Freetown that happened in 1999, he sent his family to another village. When the rebels stormed the city, Patrick became trapped at his father-in-law's house along with 150 others.

Yelling threats of death and maiming, the rebel force began burning houses, forcing out those in hiding. Patrick could hear the screams of the ones caught, knowing the rebels were cutting off their hands. As they came closer and closer to the house where Patrick and the others hid, a woman on the street began to put up a loud ruckus. The rebels, distracted, moved on, missing the house and all those in it, sparing Patrick and all with him.

That was the story Patrick told us when he arrived in 2002 for his long-awaited follow-up surgery. The very next year, when we returned, he underwent his fourth and final operation; his transformation finally fully complete.

Sierra Leone itself, however, was another thing. Already classified as the poorest nation of the world, the country was literally in a shambles, decimated by war. The vision of Mercy Ships had always been to go where we were most needed. So, in the years ahead, we made a commitment to Sierra Leone. It would become a place we returned to again and again, and then, after the turn of the century, a place where we chose to have a full-time presence.

Meanwhile, the other side of the globe was not without its Mercy Ships drama as well. All through the late 1980s and early 1990s, the *Good Samaritan* had been serving the Caribbean in relief and medical outreach efforts. She had even made one trip to the South Pacific and one to the edge of the African continent, as well as two trips to South America. Her crew took her up the Amazon River taking dentists into villages far inland. The 'Little Giant' also had a brush with worldwide athletic fame. The US Olympic Committee paid to renovate the ship, enabling her for service to the Pan American Games in Havana, Cuba. The *Good Samaritan* was the first vessel in thirty years to sail from America to communist Cuba with US governmental permission.

But the 'Little Giant' just wasn't big enough for the dream we had of a floating eye-surgery hospital for the Caribbean and Central America. So in 1995, we bought a Norwegian coastal cruise ship, renamed it the *Caribbean Mercy* and began transforming it into the floating eye hospital of our Mercy Ships dreams. The 'Good Sam' was just the right size for ports in the South Pacific. We renamed the ship the *Island Mercy* and moved it into service there to join the *Pacific Ruby*, a small donated yacht used for relief work in the South Pacific area for a short time during the early 1990s.

The *Island Mercy* was right at home in the South Pacific. In 1999, for instance, the crew treated more than twenty-four thousand patients in six nations from Tonga to the Philippines, partnering with local groups in new and wonderful ways.

In Gilligan City, Philippines, for example, the local Kiwanis Club had pre-screened a group of the region's neediest people for dental and optical assessments, and local dentists and opticians had joined the *Island Mercy* crew to help meet the demand. While in Manila, during the same Philippine visit, the ship's crew also saw 135 Filipinos a day during a medical outreach with people who lived in the city's garbage dumps. This type of service would become the norm for the little Mercy Ship.

Meanwhile, the *Caribbean Mercy*, Mercy Ships' newest fleet member, performed its initial act of mercy before it even docked at its first port. On the way to her first medical assignment in the Dominican Republic, with a new crew of eighty-one, including several families, the *Caribbean Mercy* sailed not only into bad weather and high seas, but also into the path of history.

About eight miles off the northeast coastline of Cuba, in whitecap waves, one of the crew sighted a small boat in distress. The people in

Crew of the *Africa Mercy* and the *Anastasis* meet when the two ships dock side by side in the UK.

En route to South Korea and the Philippines,
the *Caribbean Mercy* crew enjoyed spectacular scenery as the Mercy
Ships navigated the Inside Passage in Alaska.

As many as five thousand people wait patiently for a chance of life-changing surgery in Sierra Leone.

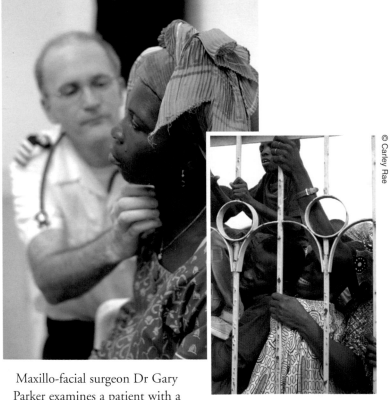

Maxillo-facial surgeon Dr Gary Parker examines a patient with a goiter to see if she can be selected as a surgical candidate for an onboard operation.

An estimated 5,000-6,000 desperate Togolese people wait to be screened.

Former Mercy Ships Captain Clem Ketchum carries a child from the surgery ward onboard one of our hospital ships.

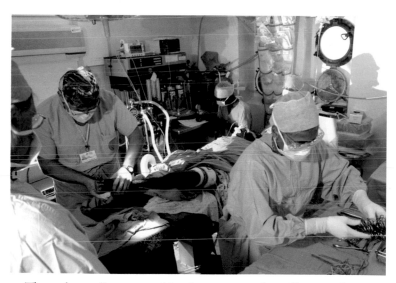

The orthopaedic team working in a compact but efficient onboard theatre while docked in Sierra Leone, the world's poorest country.

Nine-year-old Edoh could barely eat due to the tumour that destroyed her nose and filled her mouth. As the growth was blocking her airway, Edoh was also at risk of suffocation.

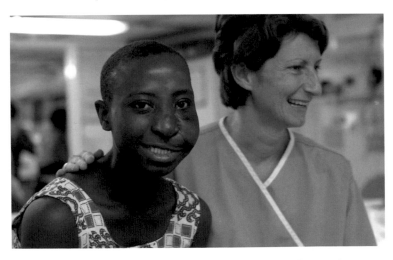

Dr Gary Parker and Dr Luer removed the tumour and created an eye socket, a roof for her mouth and a new nose. Two more surgeries were later performed and Edoh now looks forward to finishing school so that she can become a nurse and help others.

Patrick lived with this tumour for over 15 years, enduring ridicule and rejection.

Patrick had his first onboard operation in 1992. He is now married with three children and serves as an Associate Pastor of a church in Freetown.

Ten-year-old Isabelle was born in El Salvador with severe clubfeet. She learned to 'walk' on the tops of her feet, dragging herself from place to place. The object of cruel teasing, Isabelle scarcely lifted her head. Dr Tim Jones spent many hours in the operating room to correct and turn her feet in the right direction.

After days of prolonged labour due to obstructed delivery during childbirth, three million African women are incontinent because of an obstetric fistula. Without a corrective surgery, they will leak urine continually. Embarrassed, ashamed and abandoned by their families, these women have little hope.

After surgery and recovery, these ladies, wearing 'garments of praise', celebrate with singing and dancing in the ward.

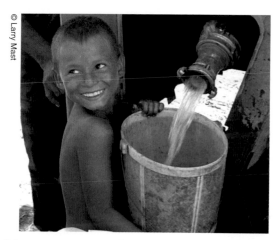

One of the greatest causes of preventable disease today is the lack of portable water. Mercy Ships well drilling teams provide clean drinking water to villages and bring a smile to a little boy's face in Nicaragua.

A focus of the work in Sierra Leone is providing mobility for people handicapped during the civil war or afflicted with polio. Individuals have been provided with prostheses, physical therapy and wheelchairs.

Mercy Ships Founder/President Don Stephens caught in a downpour in
Benin and taking the opportunity to meet locals.

Ann Gloag, Mercy Ships Director and sponsor of the *Africa Mercy*,
meets Benin President Mathieu Kerekou. From left to right: Ann Gloag,
Lord McColl, Deyon Stephens, Don Stephens and President Kerekou.

the boat were frantically waving for help. Their boat was taking on water. The captain of the *Caribbean Mercy* immediately radioed the US Coast Guard, asking for permission to help. When the Coast Guard gave the okay, the Mercy Ship moved as close to the boat as possible and pulled the people onboard just before it sank.

Over the next twenty-four hours, as the *Caribbean Mercy* continued slowly eastward against buffeting winds, the crew cared for the twenty-four people who explained they were Cuban refugees trying to escape to the United States. The next afternoon, a Coast Guard vessel arrived, and took the refugees into their charge.

This wouldn't be the last time the *Caribbean Mercy* would find itself drawn into the drama of historical events. Just a few months later, the Mercy Ship partnered with a humanitarian group to carry a cargo of high-protein food especially made for the needs of malnourished people in Haiti. On Christmas Eve 1994, we made a short stop at the port of Gonaives, Haiti, to deliver the food, supplies, and aid to a local orphanage and hospital.

United States military troops were stationed in Haiti on a peacekeeping mission at that time, following a political revolt. The entire country was in a state of civil war and economic chaos that resulted in the infamous Haiti 'boat people' refugee crisis. United States Army paratroopers from Fort Bragg, North Carolina, were stationed in Gonaives, and several of the soldiers patrolled the dock area where the *Caribbean Mercy* was located. On Christmas Day, eight of the soldiers came onboard to enjoy an evening dinner and special Christmas programme with the crew. One of the soldiers was army Sergeant Greg Cardott, who seemed to especially connect with the crew, a mutual bonding that he mentioned in letters to his wife.

Just two weeks after the ship left Haiti, Sergeant Cardott was killed while manning a highway checkpoint near Gonaives, the only American soldier to die in the entire peacekeeping mission. Nine months later, the crew of the *Caribbean Mercy*, knowing the ship would be docked at a port for a short time near Fort Bragg, invited his widow and two daughters to spend a weekend onboard. In October 1995, Greg's widow, a registered nurse, along with his daughters, spent time onboard while the ship was docked at Morehead City, North Carolina. The crew wanted to get to know her, and she wanted to know them.

The *Caribbean Mercy* soon began following the same yearly pattern as her big sister, the *Anastasis*. The ship would spend several months in the United States for maintenance and fund-raising in order to spend the rest of the year in the Caribbean basin and Central America. Each year the ship served the Caribbean's neediest residents, in nations that partnered with us, such as the Dominican Republic, Nicaragua, El Salvador, Guatemala, Honduras, and Haiti, establishing local friendships and professional relationships with government agencies and medical, charitable, humanitarian, and religious organisations on land.

What was a typical *Caribbean Mercy* port call like? A good example might be one of our visits to El Salvador. If you could have a bird's-eye view of the ship, you'd see short-term volunteer crew heading down the gangway into the city and countryside. Orthopaedic surgeons would be headed to the hospital in La Union, optometrists to the nearby army base, and Health Care Teams ferried to the nearby islands by the navy. The Health Care Teams would include audiologists fitting hearing aids, well-drillers searching for water, and dentists looking for cavities. Back onboard, you would see ophthalmologists preparing to operate, and maybe you'd catch a glimpse of the President and First Lady of El Salvador visiting the ship.

Through the years, we have had many distinguished persons visit our floating eye hospital. The President and First Lady of El Salvador have been guests. The First Lady of the Republic of Honduras, Doña

Mary Flake de Flores, visited the *Caribbean Mercy* three times during one port call. I recall her participation in one of those special moments when the bandages come off and a blind person suddenly sees – the kind I'd first experienced in Lazaros Cardenas. During her visit to the recovery room, the First Lady had asked one of the patients if she might be the one to remove the patient's eye patch. He had enthusiastically agreed. Slowly she had peeled away the patch, and the face of the First Lady of his country was the first image the patient saw.

In 2004, the new First Lady of the Republic of Honduras, Doña Aguas Ocaña de Maduro, who played a major role in the *Caribbean Mercy* return visit to Honduras, flew in by helicopter for a special reception. When she left, she took along a little girl and her mother in the helicopter to seek specialised medical treatment for the girl's facial tumour.

An amazing *Caribbean Mercy* success story is that of Isabelle. In 1999, as part of the medical outreach team that regularly goes into a port city's hospitals for screenings and subsequent surgeries, orthopaedic surgeon and Mercy Ships career crew member Dr Tim Browne met little Isabelle. Ten-year-old Isabelle had been brought to the El Salvador screening from a little village two hours away, because of her feet. Born with both feet turned completely backward, she had never been able to walk or wear shoes. To get around, Isabelle dragged herself on the tops of her feet. Working together with local surgeons, after several surgeries, Dr Browne eventually managed to turn Isabelle's feet the normal direction.

As you might imagine, the 'before' and 'after' pictures show an astounding change. But for Isabelle, wearing shoes was the most astounding change. When the Mercy Ship was back in El Salvador the very next year, a team paid a follow-up visit to see how Isabelle was doing. The team travelled to her little village and found Isabelle doing well. They discovered, though, that she had a baby sister who was just learning to walk on clubfeet. The team made arrangements for Isabelle's little sister to be operated on as well.

In 2001, while the ship was docked in Guatemala, the *Caribbean Mercy* experienced an earthquake to rival the *Anastasis'* experience in Greece. Working in a tropical weather zone, never knowing what might happen next, the ship's holds are usually kept as full of emergency supplies as possible. So, when the ground suddenly shook, and the sea began to rock and roll under the ship, the ship was ready to help.

The crew learned that the epicentre was in neighbouring El Salvador. Hundreds were killed, and hundreds of thousands were left homeless. A medical team from the ship sprang into action. Assembling supplies on hand, the crew returned to El Salvador to join the relief efforts, where aftershocks continued while they helped the injured and homeless.

Part of our crew's routine involved speaking at health clinics on shore, and where there was no clinic, sometimes to pitch in with the locals and build one. Homes, churches, clinics, wells, orphanages, latrines – Mercy Ships' short-term volunteer crew, bringing their expertise along with them, have built them all. With such talent, we began setting up land-based resource and support offices around the world, including a permanent land base in Nicaragua and in Sierra Leone.

With each passing year, the world began to feel smaller. We began to dream of filling the oceans with a fleet of sea-going ships of mercy. We began to think big, not just in possibilities, but also in size. For the work we were doing, we decided that all future Mercy Ships should be as big as the *Anastasis*. We needed more operating rooms to allow for more operations at each port stay, more recovery rooms, more rooms for the crew – more room for more of everything.

So by the turn of the century, we made plans to say goodbye to the *Island Mercy* and *Pacific Ruby*, and throw all our resources into acquiring ships big enough to take in our growing vision. We began to brainstorm plans for this new growing fleet idea – an *Africa Mercy*, an *Asia Mercy*, and an *Atlantic Mercy*. And as we were just beginning to envision such ships, out of the blue we received an invitation from the North Korean embassy representative in Switzerland to bring the *Caribbean Mercy* to their country.

Historically we knew the development of new contacts for Mercy Ships was linked to a visit of a ship, so we accepted, seeing this perhaps as a first step towards an Asian Mercy Ship. We made plans to specialise in eye surgeries, train some of the North Korean eye surgeons in new techniques, provide a million dollars' worth of new surgical equipment, and bring rice and relief materials. The protocol was signed, and soon we were en route.

We brought the *Caribbean Mercy* through the Panama Canal up the Pacific coast of Central America, towards Alaska. From Seattle we sailed on the inside passage to Seward, Kodiak Island, with short stops in Petropavlovsk, Russia. We sailed through ten time zones and seven bodies of water, and just as we were within one hundred miles of North Korea, we were notified that the conditions of our invitation were rescinded. Only days before, vessels from North and South Korea had engaged in an incident over territorial fishing water rights. North and South Korea navies exchanged fire, and thirty North Koreans were killed.

The North Korean government, although they had previously agreed to waive all port charges and welcome us, now told us they had changed their minds. They now wanted to charge us ten thousand dollars a day port fees with no guarantee as to when the ship would be offloaded or how long we would have to stay. Immediately we could see a scenario where this could become a financial nightmare, or worse. We feared that the ship, albeit on a mission of charity, might become a hostage in the middle of this dispute.

So we made the decision not to continue the voyage to North Korea. Sadly, we sailed instead for Dalian, China, where we offloaded our supplies and transferred them to a partner charity that would send the goods to help the people of Vietnam.

However, one moment in our visit to Dalian reminded me again of the need for an *Asia Mercy* ship. I met with the Chinese delegate to the World Health Organisation during that time. We were discussing the *Caribbean Mercy*'s eye-surgery expertise when I mentioned the often quoted World Health Organisation's statistic of 60 million needy blind in the world. I'll never forget her response:

'We have done the best we can to get statistics, but we all realise we could have 60 million blind in China alone. There is ample opportunity for us to partner with you and your ship right here.'

And so we continue to dream.

After three months in South Korea, laying the groundwork for a future Mercy Ship for Asia, the *Caribbean Mercy* took the opportunity to sail into the Philippines for a historic meeting with the *Island Mercy* and a medical-assignment partnership in Pulupandan, Philippines, before sailing back via Manila to its Caribbean basin home. A local marching band in brightly coloured uniforms greeted us – a marvellous sight after the North Korean experience, to say the least.

When we came close, the *Island Mercy* blew her horn and sent up five flares, much to our delight. We learned that to enable the bigger *Caribbean Mercy* to come into port, the island's dredger had to work overtime to make the channel deep enough, and had broken down twice in as many days. But soon the two sister ships were berthed side by side, performing eye surgeries on the *Caribbean Mercy* and running a dental clinic onboard the *Island Mercy*.

By the turn of a new century, the Mercy Ships had grown into a

34 million dollar per year non-profit hospital ship charity with offices in seventeen nations, a growing fleet, and an international board reflecting the diverse background and expertise of our crew. We had become Mercy Ships International. We all knew it was finally time for the next ship – something bigger, newer, state of the art; a ship to take us into the next chapter of Mercy Ships, to begin planning the fleet of our dreams.

But what happened next surprised us all.

ANGEL OF MERCY

PR Newswire Association, Inc, 2002

 Headline: Ann Gloag: Angel of Mercy
Dateline: London, Edinburgh, Glasgow, Los Angeles

Ann Gloag is a volunteer on a one-of-a-kind floating hospital Mercy Ship on which she helps with a mop and a broom. There are other volunteers with similar chores. So what is so unusual about Ms Gloag doing these necessary menial chores? She is the richest woman in Scotland, one of the wealthiest in the UK and founder of the multi-million pound Stagecoach Empire.

Ms Gloag, a former nurse, has become a guardian angel of Mercy, donating 4 million pounds, the biggest donation Mercy Ships has received in its history, to help build a Mercy Ship.

The Africa Mercy is the first addition in a proposed new plan to add ships to the existing fleet of floating hospitals that visit more than seventy ports worldwide, providing free medical and surgical procedures that bring health, hope, and training to people who would never be able to afford such services . . .

SHIP'S LOG: 2000–2004

Newcastle, England
$55^0 2'$ N $1^0 42'$ W

CHAPTER 11
HEADLINES TELL THE STORY

The quality of mercy it is twice blessed: It blesseth him that gives and him that takes. – *Merchant of Venice* by WILLIAM SHAKESPEARE

'Dame Norma Major to Christen New Mercy Ship!' read the headline.

From around the world, we travelled to the Newcastle shipyard on the River Tyne to stand at the edge of a dock. The Naming Ceremony of the *Africa Mercy*, the newest member of the Mercy Ships fleet, had just begun.

'I am delighted to be standing here with you as we celebrate the many voyages of hope and healing that lie ahead. It now gives me great pleasure to name this ship the *Africa Mercy*. May God bless her, and all who sail on her,' said Dame Norma Major, wife of former British Prime Minister John Major. Then she shot a champagne bottle from a launcher, the bottle smashed against the side of the ship, and the master of ceremonies of the shipyard led the crowd in three cheers as a bagpipe band began to play.

Why the bagpipes? In honour of Ann Gloag, the Scottish woman who had made the day possible.

This day was a wonderful surprise to us all. Our strategic planning, our vision for the future, called for a new fleet of Mercy Ships – one for every continent. Only recently had we decided the time was right for the first new ship. Our flagship, the *Anastasis*, was more than fifty years old. The ship was extremely well built. But even if it stayed afloat forever, the need in Africa was so great that we knew an *Africa*

Mercy was the next logical addition to our fleet. We also knew that buying a big ship was going to be much more expensive this time around, so we began meeting people and courting corporations, hoping to build up a healthy bank balance towards the purchase.

Then, in 1998, we met a woman who had already researched us, having come to the same conclusions as we had about the value of floating hospitals. We also discovered that she had investigated us with the same attention to detail that had made her one of the UK's most successful businesswomen. For Mercy Ships that was a very good thing. She pored over our annual audit and met administrators, surgeons, and board members. Finally, she found we embodied 'precisely the qualities necessary for running a successful business, the sheer efficiency of the operation, and the low cost of the delivery of the service,' as she put it.

Gloag, trained in nursing, first became interested in Africa when her company began operating bus services in Malawi and Kenya. During her early years as a nurse, she'd worked in a burns unit and was shocked to discover that African children with untreated superficial burns were dying from infections. So for several years she supplied and supported a burns unit at a hospital in the country, even after the Stagecoach bus company ceased operations there.

As she told the *Telegraph* magazine in 2001, that experience had made her acutely aware of the problems inherent in providing health care in developing nations. Surgeons she brought to the hospital were not able to operate because surgical instruments were missing or stolen, or because the electricity or water wasn't working. 'But a ship that sailed in fully equipped and which is effective from the day that it docks just struck me as the way forward.'

I'll never forget the moment she told us what she'd already decided. I had just met her. In August 1998, the *Anastasis* was docked at London and I'd invited her onboard for a tour. At the end of it, Ann turned to me and said, 'I'll buy your next ship.' I couldn't believe I'd heard what I thought I'd heard. She must have seen the look on my face, because she repeated it:

'I'll buy your next ship.'

I was speechless.

Since then, Ann has joined her world-class enthusiasm and world-wide contacts with us, to raise the 52 million dollars necessary to purchase, renovate, and equip the next ship. She has also joined the executive committee of the International Board, and become actively involved in fund-raising, budgets, and strategic planning.

In short order, we found a Danish ferry that had the space and the promise of a hospital ship of our dreams. We bought it, moved it to the British shipyard, and began the fund-raising needed to transform the huge ship into the *Africa Mercy*, scheduled to sail by 2005.

In 2002, when Mercy Ships leaders were invited to the inauguration of Benin's President Mathieu Kérékou, Ann travelled with us and stayed for two weeks serving on the ship in the hospital ward. She also found herself stuck in the mud with the rest of us, on our way to visit a village health clinic, pushing our four-wheel vehicles out of the mud during a downpour. She told us she loved every minute.

During the past few years, the transformation of Mercy Ships into a global charity has inspired many headlines, but even the quieter events were headline material to us. Hundreds of wonderful daily news events added up to big news for us at Mercy Ships International.

A sampling of those headlines tells the story of this new chapter as we sail into the future:

GREAT SCOT! IT'S MERCY SHIPS!!

'Volunteers Receive Charity Award in Home Nation of Scotland,' read the headline. Mercy Ships seems to have been blessed with great Scots at pivotal moments in our transformation. And we weren't the only ones who noticed. Scotland's leading newspaper, Glasgow's *Sunday Mail*, honoured Ann Gloag and Lord Ian McColl as recipients of their nation's 2002 Great Scot Award, for their charity involvement on behalf of Mercy Ships. Readers nominate unsung heroes for the award that has become nationally known as 'Scotland's People's Oscar'.

> Scotland's richest businesswoman, Ann Gloag, donated 4 million pounds to purchase a Mercy Ship for the global charity of Mercy Ships and is a passionate supporter of the cause. Professor The Lord McColl, top surgeon at Guy's Hospital in London, is the charity's UK spokesman and Vice Chairman of the International Board of Mercy Ships. Both Gloag and McColl currently donate significant amounts of their time and energies towards raising awareness and funding for the completion of the newest vessel in the growing Mercy Ships fleet, the *Africa Mercy*. Both Scots describe Mercy Ships as 'good value'.

These two great Scots are symbolic of the many special people, within our truly international scope, who have come onboard with Mercy Ships and are reshaping it with cyclone force – and making headlines as they do.

MERCY SHIPS TO PARTNER WITH WORLD'S LEADING TEACHING HOSPITALS

In March of 2004, Lord McColl was invited to do grand rounds at Harvard Medical School and Brigham and Women's Hospital. Lord McColl, besides being chairman of the board of the UK Mercy Ships and Vice Chairman of Mercy Ships International, has been the physician to heads of state. While at Harvard, he gave a PowerPoint presentation of some of the surgeries that we do on Mercy Ships.

Afterwards, one of the hospital's top medical educators asked an unexpected question: 'Might our residents spend some time with you on your ships? The pathology that they could be exposed to would take a lifetime to replicate here in the West.'

It was true. Lord McColl's colleagues at the teaching hospital saw something we could not. We could teach as well as heal. The developed world had totally eradicated many of the diseases and medical problems we were seeing.

At almost the same time, the University of San Francisco Children's Hospital approached us about a similar arrangement, as did Guy's Hospital, London. Would we at Mercy Ships find a way for their residents to come to serve with us?

Can you imagine how I felt when I heard this news? Talk about a win/win situation. At the time of writing, we are working on such partnerships with some of the world's most renowned teaching hospitals.

MERCY SHIPS ANNOUNCES
SATELLITE COMMUNICATIONS FOR FLEET

Communications is always a challenge on a ship. Now, though, it's rarely a problem at all for our growing fleet. Between state-of-the-art systems offered to us at cost from two leading maritime communications companies, MTN and Petrocom, we now have full-time satellite communication capabilities both in port and at sea.

But there are more reasons to be excited about this news than just ship-to-shore calls. Not only does this give us the twenty-four hour connection to the outside world we have long needed, but it also opens up a whole new dimension to the quality of care we offer in the operating rooms. Now, when surgeons onboard encounter a case they have never seen and they need to know its pathology, we consult by satellite. With a digital camera and new communications technology we can snap an image, e-mail it to, say, Harvard Medical School for a specialist's opinion on problematic cases, and in a matter of hours our surgeons can be given world-class consultation on how to treat their patients. The satellites allow a 21st century synergy like nothing else we've ever experienced, offering a level of medical care and expertise to rival any on the globe.

MATCHING GRANT OF $10 MILLION
GIVEN BY ANONYMOUS FOUNDATION

In 2002, we received a challenge we excitedly accepted to make the transformation of the *Africa Mercy* happen – a ten-million-dollar grant that would be ours if we were able to match it by raising another ten million dollars. This was a blast of great news for us, and it was an even bigger and better blast when we matched it by 2004. And headlines like the following helped it happen:

MERCY SHIPS RECEPTION HELD
AT HOUSE OF LORDS

and

FORMER PRIME MINISTER TO HOLD
NEWS CONFERENCE FOR GLOBAL CHARITY

Prominent British leaders in medicine and politics have magnanimously offered their time to further the cause of Mercy Ships International in both the UK and the US. Two such moments happened within a year of each other. In September 2002, Lord McColl hosted a reception at the House of Lords. Approximately 135 guests attended the event. The guests learned more about the work of Mercy Ships from Lord McColl, the current chairman of the UK board of trustees, and other Mercy Ships leaders. And in April 2003, former British Prime Minister John Major returned to our Texas headquarters as the guest of Mercy Ships. The prime minister spoke on behalf of Mercy Ships in the Dallas–Fort Worth area.

CREW BRINGS RELIEF TO ABANDONED SHIP

In February 2004, a Mercy Ship once again came to the rescue of people stranded at sea. As the crew of the *Anastasis* screened patients, scheduled surgeries, and set up programmes in Sierra Leone, rumours of an offshore fugitive ship with an abandoned crew and a dead captain piqued their curiosity.

After hearing talk of serious malaria cases onboard the purported fugitive ship, the *M/V Panciu*, the captain of the *Anastasis* found out via web research that the ship had changed names several times. The ship had been detained at least once in ports of call, which seemed to point to 'nefarious activity', as the captain put it. And now the crew seemingly had been abandoned so far out to sea that they couldn't help themselves.

The Mercy Ships captain gained permission from the port to do a 'humanitarian visit'; and he, along with a small contingent of crew, crossed the waters on the ship's launch carrying a few medicines and some food. They found no malaria, but the crew – all from India, Pakistan, or Bangladesh – were almost out of food and fresh water. They also hadn't been paid for eighteen months, and had little prospect of returning to their home countries.

During the next few weeks, when there was time, *Anastasis* deckhands took trips out to the ship to check on the crew. The Mercy Ships captain wrote a letter to the port authorities, helping the abandoned crew get in touch with the International Trade Workers Federation. Weeks later, the crew gratefully received pay and tickets home.

JEBBEH NOW IS SAVED!

CT SCANNER DONATED THROUGH VOLUNTEER'S BENEFIT CONCERTS

All our medical moments feel like headlines to us. The two headlines above appeared in print and are perfect examples of the impact one Mercy Ships surgical volunteer can have.

As the number of international medical experts volunteering for Mercy Ships assignments has grown, the ways that word of their work has spread back to their countries and turned into action flowing back to us has been a phenomenal thing to watch.

When maxillofacial surgeon Dr Luer Köper could not arrange for four-year-old Jebbeh to undergo surgery in Germany, he brought the surgeons to her in Sierra Leone. Dr Köper first examined Jebbeh in December 2002. The girl was born with an encephalocele, caused by a hole in the skull bones. Children born with this problem die young when meningitis inevitably sets in. Jebbeh was scheduled for a free surgery onboard the Mercy Ship, but her appointment had to be postponed for lack of time.

'I promised her we would come again and she would have a surgery onboard the ship,' Dr Köper said. Meanwhile, Dr Köper e-mailed the charity branch of AWD, a Germany economic company that offered funds to take a team of surgeons to Jebbeh. The story of Dr Köper and Jebbeh was featured in the German newspaper *Bild Am Sonntag*. A retired German journalist saw the coverage and offered to raise funds through a photography exhibition for the remaining cost of Jebbeh's operation. Finally, more than a year after Jebbeh first visited the Mercy Ship, she underwent a successful seven-hour onboard operation. Days later, a German newspaper ran the story with the headline, 'Jebbeh Now Is Saved!'

Dr Köper also noticed that the *Anastasis* was performing its medical miracles without the aid of its own CT scanner. Patients had to be sent to hospitals on land, sometimes into the next country, when surgeons needed a scanner to help in their diagnostic decisions. Even then, the scanners didn't always function properly. So, back home, Dr Köper organised two benefit concerts for the purchase of a refurbished scanner, and in July 2002 it arrived onboard. We put it to use immediately.

MERCY SHIPS DOCTOR PERFORMS REVOLUTIONARY EYE SURGERY ONBOARD

In April 2003, onboard the *Caribbean Mercy* docked at the Dominican Republic, Dr Glenn Strauss – associate of Heaton Eye Clinic and new director of health care for Mercy Ships, and a pioneer in a new type of eye surgery – performed a procedure known as conductive keratoplasty™ for the first time ever in a developing nation. The revolutionary painless and quick procedure was performed in selected US sites. For the first time, this world-class treatment was also offered to the poor in the Dominican Republic.

With our emphasis on eye surgery in the Americas and the Caribbean, this operation is a perfect example of the deepening medical partnerships we are creating with top medical consultants all over the world. As Dr Strauss put it, the procedure was a tremendous Caribbean basin opportunity to 'meet the practical vision needs of people who can't get glasses'.

CORPORATE PARTNERS INVIGORATE MERCY SHIPS' PROWESS!

JOHNSON & JOHNSON GIVES ORTHOPAEDIC SUPPLIES WORTH MILLIONS

OPHTHALMIC LASER TECHNOLOGY PROVIDED TO SERVE POOR

HEATON EYE ASSOCIATES TO DONATE ANAESTHESIA MACHINE

KIMBERLY-CLARK LENDS A HAND TO MERCY SHIPS

ALCON EMPLOYEES GIVE DAY OFF TO CREATE MERCY SHIPS PACKETS

One of the biggest reasons for our success as a hospital ship charity has been our partnership with the corporations who manufacture the medical equipment and materials that make modern medicine so successful. I am a firm believer in the synergy between the corporate world and the charitable. The two need each other. The ways that companies, made up of people like you and me, have begun to partner with us is definitely headline material.

Johnson & Johnson, for instance, has selected Mercy Ships as one of their charities of choice. It has been one of our most successful relationships. In one year alone, they donated $3 million worth of orthopaedic supplies. Hundreds of other generous corporations have made our growing errands of medical mercy around the globe not only possible, but economically feasible.

Donations are essential, but sometimes the people who make the products jump in to partner in unique and creative ways. One such story concerns the workers of Alcon, the world's leading eye care company and a major donor of surgical and pharmaceutical ophthalmic products to Mercy Ships almost from the beginning. When a Mercy Ship docked near Alcon's Houston facility, Vice President and General Manager Sally Wilson took the opportunity to tour the ship. What she saw gave her an idea.

Normally, crew members have to open many donated packets for the exact supplies needed for the Mercy Ship's most commonly performed eye surgery. Wilson thought of a way, with the help of Alcon employees, that the ship's surgeons could use their donations more efficiently. Soon, Alcon employees were enthusiastically volunteering their time to assemble the essential products into a CustomPak Kit designed specifically for Mercy Ships' special use. Now when Mercy Ships surgeons operate, they open one packet that contains everything they need. The time saved by this inspired idea allows Mercy Ships surgeons to do more eye surgeries in the time available.

CHARITY NAVIGATOR GIVES MERCY SHIPS ITS HIGHEST RATING FOUR STARS

In 2002, we were surprised to receive a notice that we had been rated by *Charity Navigator,* a charity comparison web site. *Charity Navigator* is an independent charity evaluator, heralded and recognised by publications and entities as diverse as *Reader's Digest,* CNN, the *New York Times, Christian Science Monitor,* and the

Washington Post. The news was good: Mercy Ships was placed in *Charity Navigator's* highest category for efficiency and vision. They described us as blurring the lines between 'previously discrete domains of profits and philanthropy, business and social concerns'. Value-based living that 'integrates personal and professional concerns is the key to future impact', it went on to say. The summary added:

> Mercy Ships begins as the story of hardy visionaries retooling an ocean liner to bring medical help to the neediest locales around the world. That essential passion is unchanged. Men and women actually pay for the privilege of living in cramped quarters on a floating city with other volunteers from scores of nations. Some use accumulated wealth, others raise support as charitable staff. All participants, from swabbies to surgeons, have a sense of purpose and job satisfaction that Franklin-Covey (in a recent professional review) rates as among the highest ever encountered.
>
> (Source: www.charitynavigator.org)

That description of the evolution of our first quarter-century captures the spirit of Mercy Ships remarkably well – what we have been, what we want to be, and what we are and always will be.

MERCY SHIPS VISION AWARDS GALA HELD IN WASHINGTON, DC

In 2002, Mercy Ships hosted a Vision Awards Gala in Washington, DC, one of the many special opportunities we have had to spend time with leaders of both the developed and developing world who have embraced Mercy Ships' unique charitable vision. That night, we honoured the humanitarian efforts of people such as the former First Lady of the Republic of Honduras Mary Flake de Flores; Anthony Hall, US ambassador to the World Food Programme in Rome; Daniel Snyder, owner of the NFL Washington Redskins, whose philanthropic organisation has gathered more than forty local area businesses to benefit causes such as handicapped children's efforts, literacy, educational and sports programmes; and CNN talk show host Larry King whose personal foundation 'The Larry King Cardiac Foundation' helps people who cannot afford to pay for heart disease treatment – including children from Benin, West Africa.

Paying special tribute to such visionaries was memorable. But I also recall the night for its unique sense of perspective. To sit at a Four Seasons Hotel with influential people in the United States' capital city immediately after a months-long Mercy Ship assignment in the world's poorest nation was an odd sensation. And yet it's one I've experienced many times, because such a scenario makes perfect sense from a Mercy Ships point of view. The capacity and desire for mercy in those of us most blessed is the same as that of the people who most need it. And Mercy Ships International's unique and special mission is to be a floating bridge between the two worlds.

And that vision, now in the shape of the 16,000-ton new *Africa Mercy*, doubling the medical mercy we can offer the African continent, inspires us to keep dreaming for the day when there will be a Mercy Ship for every continent and we will have the privilege of filling the oceans with mercy.

MERCY SHIPS BEGINS TO DREAM OF REACHING ONE MILLION PEOPLE A YEAR

A million people a year served by a Mercy Ship – that's our goal. For Mercy Ships International, truly the best is yet to come, as we bring hope and healing to the ends of the earth and back again. With the help of just such newsworthy partnerships as these, we hope to be making a million headlines in a million personal lives as we continue to keep sailing, and as we begin also to find our way down the gangway and onto land.

THE STORY OF AMINATA AND SANDY

 Dateline: Freetown, Sierra Leone
8°30' N 13°15' W

'I had everything I needed,' said the forty-something year old. 'It was time to give something back.' So Sandy volunteered with Mercy Ships. She worked in the ship's reception. By day, she answered phones, fielded questions, averted catastrophes. By night, she headed to the ward to spend time with her first African friend, Aminata. Only ten years separated the two women. They liked to talk and laugh. They were both independent, brave, industrious. There, though, the similarities ended. Sandy owned her own home. Aminata owned barely more than the clothes on her back. Sandy had health, financial security, many friends. Aminata was sick, indigent, friendless.

Aminata was called 'the witch of Freetown' because of a tumour the size of a grapefruit growing on the side of her jaw. She lost her husband, her friends, her business in clothing retail. She turned to making money as best she could – peeling oranges for sale on the side of the street. One night she dreamed of a hospital ship that would heal her. Months later, a Mercy Ship docked in Freetown. Soon, surgeons removed Aminata's tumour and inserted a titanium jaw implant. Aminata stayed weeks onboard the ship – to Sandy's delight.

Sandy served with Mercy Ships for eight years before returning home. Ten years after she first met Aminata, Sandy made a surprise trip to Sierra Leone. One of her goals was to see Aminata again, and soon the two were laughing and talking like old times. Aminata, now reconciled with her husband, returned home bearing gifts from Sandy.

Sandy returned home convinced of three facts – friendships shape our lives; giving has its own reward; and it is possible to make a difference in a world of need.

SHIP'S LOG: 2000–2005

Brikama, The Gambia
13°27' N 16°35' W

CHAPTER 12

MERCY SHIPS ON LAND AND SEA

He is no fool who gives what he cannot keep to gain what he cannot lose. – JIM ELLIOTT

On a street named Mercy Ships Avenue, we're in the middle of a celebration.

The nation's Vice President, hundreds of villagers and local clinic workers, and crew members were all together for the day-long opening ceremony of a brand-new, just finished HIV/AIDS clinic. And as a lasting tribute to the dedicated crew who guided it into existence, the grateful Brikama community had named the street 'Mercy Ships Avenue'.

Our friend, Dr Gisela Schneider of WEC International, who had begun an HIV/AIDS project to battle the epidemic threatening to turn Africa into a 'continent of caskets' – as one UN official so graphically put it – had been treating her patients out of a storage closet, the only available space at the overcrowded Brikama Health Centre.

When she heard a Mercy Ship was coming to The Gambia, Dr Schneider contacted us, and our volunteer crew jumped at the opportunity to help. In only four months, Mercy Ship volunteers and local villagers, guided by our community development team, constructed two vitally needed buildings, one to be called the Brikama Health Clinic to teach reproductive health, the other to be a hospice.

'I have worked in Africa for a long time and can practise medicine in a hole in the ground or beneath the shade of a tree,' Dr Schneider said that day. 'But now I will have running water and a sink to wash my hands in. Thank you,' she said to the special crew.

If I were ever to wonder whether the Mercy Ships idea is bigger than my personal vision or touched by a providential hand, I would only have to think about the people involved and the explosion of their energy right down the gangway and onto shore.

We were already experienced in relief work and community development from the years before we began full-time hospital-ship work. These ports around the world were becoming home for our Mercy Ships and during our months-long port stays, we had growing opportunities to work onshore. Medical and dental teams established field clinics in communities near each port city to offer local people basic health care. The more we served onshore, the more we began to see ways we might help break the cycle of poverty and disease that drove thousands to a Mercy Ship for healing and help.

Could a hospital ship charity make a lasting difference on land as well?

The volunteer dynamic of Mercy Ships seemed tailor-made for such a venture. The influx of different talents and energy and diverse skills from month to month on a Mercy Ship naturally lent itself to new ideas that no poop deck could hold for long.

So, in partnership with other humanitarian and charitable organisations, we began each year to do more and more work onshore. Immediate needs always come first, just as they do onboard the ship. Sometimes we'd help build an orphanage, other times a clinic, quite often a freshwater well or a latrine. Nobody who has ever visited a developing country can deny the immediate need and health benefits of a good, dependable latrine – not to mention the skills to build and maintain it.

Of course, the more we were involved in projects on land, the more we needed to be on land. Since the ships would ultimately sail away to other ports, we soon had a critical need for follow-ups that can only be done by trained local partners, during and after Mercy Ship port visits.

As you might imagine, we began to think deeply about what a 'Mercy Ships on Land' dynamic would mean. We decided that such work would always have a Mercy Ships difference by developing an 'on land' philosophy of partnerships with local people, empowering them to make a future for themselves. Whether it's building homes, digging latrines, establishing wells, teaching health care or effective farming techniques, each project would include the education of local representatives who could train others, passing on the skills.

This had been a basic tenet of the SS *Hope,* one of our earliest inspirations for Mercy Ships. Their doctors would heal, but they'd also teach local doctors modern skills so the work could continue after the ship sailed. That's the spirit our Mercy Ships team would take with them down the gangway.

Classic thinking in the world of development says that to make a difference one must work with the big picture, the good of the many being more important than the individual. Of course, individuals such as Edoh, Tamba, Adam, Angelle, Daisy, and others you've read about in this book might strongly debate that idea.

We've decided to attempt both. A hospital ship is definitely focused on cure, but we also embrace the classic prevention idea, too. We just happen to add a Mercy Ships twist. Our focus will always be on the individual. But every group is made up of individuals, and each valued individual can serve a larger group of individuals. One person, healthy and equipped with self-sufficiency skills, has the power to change the future of his or her family. And each self-sufficient family adds to the health and welfare of its entire village.

Where Mercy Ships strategically can help this happen, we will have made a lasting difference on land as well as sea.

From the Caribbean to Africa, and back again, we have already seen such partnerships work wonders.

Let me take you on a quick trip around the world with Mercy Ships On Land.

Puerto Cortes, Honduras
15°51' N 87°57' W

ELVER AND THE SPECIAL NAIL

Gunshot and machete wounds, falls from mango trees, and injuries from hard labour provide an unending supply of battered and broken bodies to fill the orthopaedic ward at each port's 'poor man's hospital'. ER patients lie on beds, stretchers, and on the floor, often without sheets to comfort their broken bodies. It can be overwhelming, but over and again we learn that a little can always go a long way in the developing world. The story of a boy named Elver is a good example of how it's possible to battle poverty – one family at a time.

Fifteen-year-old Elver had the sole responsibility for his family after his father went to prison. On a summer day in his high mountain village of Yoro, after he'd put in a full day constructing fences on a piece of farmland, Elver had gone to the soccer field to have some fun. One false move later, and Elver had fractured his leg – badly. With money loaned by an uncle, Elver travelled for four hours in an ambulance to the nearest medical facility. Once there, things only got worse. He stayed alone for days in the overflow ward off the emergency room, stranded, because he had no money to pay for the surgery necessary to help his leg.

Mercy Ships orthopaedic surgeon Dr Lee Zirkle was visiting the hospital during the ship's Honduras stay and met Elver. He saw that

Elver's leg would never heal properly even if he could afford the surgery available. But Dr Zirkle was convinced Elver was a good candidate for something he had designed especially for use in international orthopaedic relief projects – something called a 'surgical implant generation network nail'. It worked. With Elver back on his feet, he could support his family again. Dr Zirkle is a fine example of the kind of cutting-edge medical experts who volunteer to serve on a Mercy Ship. And Elver is a fine example of how meeting the needs of the one can change the future of the many.

Cotonou, Benin
6°21' N 2°23' E

SAVING THE BABIES

When we are invited to meet village tribal chieftains or elders, we always ask them: 'What are the greatest needs you see?'

Almost invariably, the chieftain will say, 'Our children and our grandchildren are our security for our old age. But so many of our babies don't live, and we don't know what causes this. Our children seem normal, and then they die.'

It's true. Infant mortality is mind-boggling in sub-Saharan Africa – one in four children do not live to see their fifth birthday.

The major preventative solution is so simple. Unbelievably, almost 80 per cent of human illness would be eliminated from the entire planet if everyone had access to clean water and basic sanitation. Teaching basic hygiene alone can save countless babies' lives.

So, when we asked that question to the elders during our stay in Benin, we were prepared for their answer. Using creative visual methods, we explained to people who had never seen a microscope about the impact of germs, about the cycle of the hookworm and other diseases caused by poor hygiene. Mercy Ships teams have developed some very creative ways to teach this. Trust me – once you've seen the 'green hand' demonstration, you'll never forget to wash your hands again.

Using a washbasin and a hand painted green to represent germs, the teachers spread that green around everywhere and to everyone with handshakes, eating, touching, and similar actions, while being unable to wash it off using only water. That simple demonstration alone has helped countless African villages become healthier.

Simple actions such as penning animals, wearing shoes, washing hands, and cleaning the water save children's lives. With our teachers-teaching-teachers philosophy of community health education, Mercy Ships teams pass on instruction methods such as 'the green hand', so that essential health knowledge becomes part of the village's culture.

At the same time, we also build maternity-care clinics, partnering with local community leaders. Once a month, in Benin, for example, mothers can now bring their babies into the new clinic to make sure they are healthy and up-to-date with their vaccinations. To see the joy on these mothers' faces as they hold their normal, healthy children is a special joy for us. Each healthy child is one less child in danger of dying or in need of our shipboard help.

Leon, Nicaragua
12°24' N 86°52' W

Freetown, Sierra Leone
8°30' N 13°15' W

SEA LEGS AND NEW STEPS

Crew members often come up with brilliant solutions to the many problems we encounter. 'Operation Sea Legs', for instance, was an idea that ultimately inspired our first two permanent land programmes.

Staff prosthetist Paul Moehring had a brainstorm after he created an artificial leg for a West African patient. The problem of land mines left in the aftermath of wars had begun to gain global media attention. According to one recent estimate, up to one hundred million mines remain buried in sixty-seven countries. More than one hundred thousand land mines, for example, purportedly remain buried in Nicaragua – and its civil war ended in 1990.

Children playing, farmers working their fields, and innocents going about their lives step on these mines and lose limbs. Paul believed that Mercy Ships could not only help these people with custom prosthetics, we could build custom ones on the spot.

'Operation Sea Legs' had begun. Paul raised funds to buy an insulated forty-foot container, which he then fitted out over several years as a complete mobile prosthetic workshop able to produce an accurate and well-fitted leg within four to five hours. As soon as it was ready, we moved it to Nicaragua to respond to the need of land mine amputees there. After a while, it became apparent that physical rehabilitation alone was not enough to help amputees. Land mine casualties required sustained, long-term support services focused on helping victims earn a living and become better integrated into their communities.

So Operation Sea Legs changed its name in 1999 to 'New Steps', indicating a new direction for the programme. And that direction took it towards Freetown, Sierra Leone, and the land-based programme in Nicaragua broadened to encompass the support services as well as other perceived needs.

In 1999, the civil war in Sierra Leone reached the capital city, Freetown. Before the fighting was over, an estimated two thousand people in the Freetown area had lost limbs amputated by the rebel forces. Thousands more had polio, an indirect result of the war, since vaccinations ceased during the decade of conflict. Mercy Ships' New Steps programme started small, with a dedicated staff of only five, in January 2000.

In April, the prosthetic container arrived.

In May, rebel forces took 500 United Nations peacekeepers captive in the city. So the New Steps team was evacuated by UN helicopter to Guinea.

When the war finally ended, the New Steps team returned to a devastated Sierra Leone to discover that war does much more to a body than physical damage. It tears a person's heart and soul. So New Steps committed to healing lives as well as bodies, with an integrated programme that provides rehabilitation, health care, and social and economic services to thousands who have been disabled and displaced by war, land mines or disease.

Soon, New Steps was partnering with organisations such as Rotary International, Wheelchairs for the World, and the United Methodist Church to provide not only prosthetic limbs but also wheelchairs. As one woman pulled herself along the ground towards her new wheelchair, she stated, 'I will never drag myself on the ground again.' Once you hear something like that, you are never the same.

Our first permanent land-based presence, Mercy Ships Nicaragua, recently registered with the government at the highest level available for nongovernmental humanitarian agencies, and its staff is offering a host of services from short-term volunteer projects and community development programmes to organic farming.

Mercy Ships Nicaragua's goal is to contribute to the long-term development of the country and to provide a training location dedicated to preparing volunteers from both developed and developing nations to serve on future Mercy Ships projects worldwide, with a special emphasis on medical, relief, and community development experience. Both programmes, in Sierra Leone and Nicaragua, are true 'landlubber' undertakings, in business to stay.

Molambay, Sierra Leone
8°30' N 13°15' W

MERCY SHEEP

Another example of creative thinking that gives a whole new meaning to the term 'poop deck' is the 'Mercy Sheep' project. In 2002, goats and sheep were purchased in The Gambia, corralled onto the aft deck of the *Anastasis* and pampered by the crew for thirty-six hours, while sailing to Sierra Leone to replenish the livestock decimated by the country's civil war. More than 160 families in the isolated and war-devastated Molambay region outside of Freetown accepted the donated livestock and promised to donate the first female kid or lamb from the first two litters produced by their animal to a relative or neighbour, thereby helping to multiply the effort throughout the whole community.

The happy recipients of each animal had to first attend a training session with two men from the Ministry of Agriculture and a local veterinarian who helped Mercy Ships with the project. The training included the basics of proper care, feeding and watering, handling, and some information on identifying diseases. They also had to provide a shelter for their animal before receiving it and a small amount of money to cover the vaccination expenses. In 2004, Mercy Sheep volunteers hosted the country's first Sheep and Goat Show. The proud owners led their animals into an arena to be viewed in six categories. The animals were judged and prizes awarded. The local community members decided to make the show an annual event.

LATRINES, MICROCREDITS, SWORDS, AND PLOUGHSHARES

After soldiers decimated the village of Molambay, rumours spread that these Revolutionary United Front rebels had dumped dead bodies into the clean water wells as they swept through, leaving little in their wake but destruction. Farms turned to weeds and brush, houses turned to heaps, wells turned stagnant; the people had abandoned them running for their lives, not returning until the war's end.

The rumours of dead bodies in the wells caused the returning locals to abandon them, fearing what they might find inside. And while the Mercy Ship Water and Sanitation team never discovered evidence to prove the rumour true, they did find Molambay's wells in severe disrepair and sorely neglected. So the team taught a group of young men water and sanitation principles, including how to resurrect their dilapidated wells. Some of these same men have begun latrine-making businesses, marketing their skills to other villages to help provide for their families. With maintained latrines, fewer people will find themselves in the grip of the scourges that have been completely eliminated in the developed world.

If you believe in the value of the individual, treating people with dignity is of prime importance. So is breaking the cycle of poverty and dependence. Mercy Ships also has designed programmes to give small, or microcredit, loans for individual Africans to start micro-enterprises, helping to stabilise their local economy while giving people one more way to reclaim their own futures. The idea is to partner with people in the villages to establish 'cottage' industries, jumpstarting sustainable development. Some of these industries are quite remarkable.

Talk about turning swords into ploughshares – men in Calaba

Town, a suburb of Freetown, have turned Mercy Ships' New Steps microcredit loans into the creation of some very interesting products. A talented group of handicapped war and polio victims works with Father Burton, an Italian priest famous for his rehabilitation work with ex-rebel boys. They mould cast-off brass mortar shell casings into everyday utensils as well as things of beauty, such as crosses. Their group, Handicapped Action Movement, is transforming tools of war into works of art – including handsome Mercy Ship logos – winning contracts from government, local humanitarian groups, and people in the community for their skills.

We established programmes expressly for the women in the West African ports we visited. For example, along with a new dress, a new hat, and a plastic photo ID card, we give microcredit loans to women who undergo corrective VVF surgery to help them become self-sufficient.

The Women's Initiative Programme is one of these programmes. Alongside other nongovernmental agencies, Mercy Ships crew members are working to help village women become leaders in their communities. I especially love the 'princess project' which trains local women in commerce and cottage industries. Besides offering classes on family planning, pre- and postnatal practices, and women's health issues, the Women's Initiative also offers courses in sewing, tie-dyeing, soap making, knitting, bookkeeping practices, and rudimentary marketing so they can market the products that they produce.

Many villages have built earthen baking ovens so that women who had no means of economic support can make a living selling bread to their own villages, and to the surrounding villages as well. At the time of writing, clay ovens for making bread have been built in sixteen villages and are now self-supporting, having been begun with funds provided by Mercy Ships. The unmistakable mouth-watering aroma of baking bread wafts throughout the village and within hours the bread is sold out. The group shares the income among the women's families involved in the project.

Las Casitas, Nicaragua
12°42' N 86°59' W

AFTER HURRICANES AND COFFEE

Sometimes we find ourselves in the midst or aftermath of natural disasters, restoring hope and healing any way we can, as has been the case throughout our history. In 1998, not two months after the *Caribbean Mercy* crew had finished a port visit that included a medical assistance and development project at a village by the volcano Las Casitas, they were horrified to watch television coverage of Hurricane Mitch. Torrents of mud, trees, and boulders were cascading down the volcano destroying everything in their path – a path many of the crew had recently walked. The scene resembled a moonscape; nothing was left of the homes, schools, or people in its way. The crew decided to return to help as soon as possible.

In the meantime, a small team returned to the area using any mode of transportation possible. Several members of the team hitched a ride on a foreign military helicopter as they made emergency food drops to communities cut off by flooding from the immense rain, then rode the rest of the way on an army truck to the mudslide area.

The scene was horrifying. Bodies were everywhere, stuck in the mudflow. Dead people, horses, and cows littered the landscape. Those who survived told the same story. The water was rising in their village. Streets were turning into small rivers. They waited inside until they heard something that sounded like helicopters coming to help them, but what they saw instead was the entire mountain coming down. Mothers told tales of their children being ripped out of their arms by the mudflow. Survivors told of being stripped naked by the force of the mud.

Amazingly enough, the mud miraculously separated and went around several of the homes of the people the *Caribbean Mercy* team had come to know, leaving intact the two wells that Mercy Ships helped the community dig. They became the only source of clean water for miles in the wake of the disaster.

The *Caribbean Mercy* soon arrived with over $2.5 million of medical supplies and medicine for the local hospitals. Cargo holds were full; the crew cabins were full. Every available space was stuffed with goods. The crew filled their backpacks with clothes and food to give away. For three days they took two trips per day to hand out supplies to the survivors. When the ship sailed, two members stayed behind to help take remaining relief supplies farther inland.

The Hurricane Mitch emergency relief run to Nicaragua was the largest scale emergency relief undertaking in the *Caribbean Mercy*'s history and led to the creation of a permanent land-based operation in Leon.

An estimated 850,000 people were displaced during the hurricane, many of them permanently. The challenge was overwhelming, but our new land-based team launched into relief and longer-term development projects, working through local contacts and organisations, always keeping in mind Mercy Ships' belief in the importance of the individual. Soon, short-term volunteers arrived to begin conducting health clinics and well decontamination programmes. During the six months following the hurricane, Mercy Ships Nicaragua served more than 100,000 persons in several hundred rural communities affected by the hurricane. Today, in Las Casitas, a park stands in memoriam to those who perished in the volcanic mudslide.

La Palmerita, Nicaragua
12°35' N 86°40' W

El Tanque, Nicaragua
12°31' N 86°57' W

TALE OF TWO VILLAGES

After Hurricane Mitch, Nicaragua faced not only the same reconstruction needs we saw after the civil war in Sierra Leone, but the havoc of that incredible storm and its effects. Even periodic volcanic eruptions wreak havoc, spewing ash that kills crops and farm animals. So this was the moment that Mercy Ships Nicaragua came into its own. Here, as in Africa, the fundamental objective was to partner with local people, to see them ultimately become self-sufficient, helping others to help themselves. Sometimes that meant helping two communities connect with each other.

El Tanque was a community that had to start again with nothing, having been displaced by the devastating Casita mudslide in 1998. They ultimately became completely self-sufficient, even making quite a profit on the crops they grow on their land.

La Palmerita, though, was another story. In fact, it was not even a 'real' village. After many jobless and homeless farmers protested in the nation's capital demanding help following the recent crash of the coffee industry, the Nicaraguan president granted them land to begin new lives. So, 160 of these families moved to the land to create the coffee refugee community of La Palmerita.

Think about it: People from several devastated communities were suddenly thrown together to build one community where there wasn't one before. Mercy Ships Nicaragua helped with food distributions, construction, water and sanitation, health and agricultural projects, as best its team could, but the leaders saw that the community wouldn't be self-sufficient before the food distributions ceased.

So Mercy Ships Nicaragua decided to introduce the two communities – El Tanque and La Palmerita. The team set up community get-togethers, to introduce the village leaders and families, so neighbours could give advice to neighbours, helping each other and thereby helping themselves. And that is exactly what has happened.

Katigbo, Benin
6°30' N 2°47' E

THE PLACE OF DYING

I have seen what a transformation such efforts can make, with my own eyes, in only a matter of years. The transformation can be literally from death to life.

In Benin, along what is known as the 'old slave coast', is an area called Katigbo. It has one of the highest infant mortality rates, lowest life expectancies, and worst economic conditions of the entire nation, and it has been known for hundreds of years as 'the place of the dying' – the literal meaning of the word *Katigbo*.

Not too far away is 'The Road of No Return', and at its end stands the monument to the old slave-gathering castle, where captured slaves would be made to walk seven times around the castle's tree, which by legend would make the new slaves forget their past, dying to their previous lives of freedom.

As I drove along the road to Katigbo in 1998, I saw all sorts of cottage industries based around the woodworking of beautiful native teak, rosewood, and other exotic hardwoods. But what they were making were coffins – ornate, hand-carved coffins. Their beauty was heart-stopping. I saw one that looked like the head of a rooster, another like an airplane; the creativity seemed to know no bounds. Soon I learned that this was Katigbo's main industry – the building of coffins. Its people spent more money for the coffin and burial ceremony for their loved ones than they would have spent on them during the entire rest of their lives.

As I gazed at all this, I realised why. Death was still everywhere. Long after the slave trade was gone, people were still dying, but now the deaths were from rampant disease, malnutrition, and horrid economic conditions. Death was a major part of the culture. There was a pervasive lack of hope to change anything for the better, so the mourning was constant – from cradle to certain, quick grave. They knew no other way but death. It became their culture in a way we can never quite understand.

In the months ahead, along with local partnerships and with the aid of other nongovernmental groups in the country, Mercy Ships teams went into the villages along this road and began to work to break this cycle. We began to teach basic health care and hygiene lessons, and to teach suitable students how to teach others these basics. We partnered with them to build a maternity clinic to help decrease the death rate for mothers and babies.

Their land was fertile, but the villagers starved half the year, because they had no way of storing grain. So Mercy Ships teams partnered with the village leaders to build their own granaries. We helped with design and oversight; they built it, and they owned it. After the ship departed, the Beninois students trained by Mercy Ships in a district called Ifangni, fifty-five miles from Cotonou, formed a registered nongovernmental organisation, called 'D4D Anastasis'.

D4D stands for development in four dimensions – the spiritual, social, intellectual, and physical. Now under their own initiative, D4D has developed plans to build a community centre and grain storage facility to house grain during the non-growing season so their communities can counter the malnourishment their children suffer during the lean months. They pool funds and purchase grain in quantity at the lowest prices during the harvest season, sell the grain back to their community with a small surcharge to cover costs; by doing so they have seen a small profit as well as broken the cycle of malnutrition and poverty. After we sailed, we heard that the group was planning a water tower and had organised plans for construction and financing, entirely on their own.

Five years later, I returned to Benin. As I drove along the same Katigbo road, I found myself speechless at the change I saw. The main enterprise along the road was still woodworking, using the wonderful, exotic woods all ornately, beautifully crafted – but the products were now beds, chairs, tables, and furniture – things for the living.

What had changed?

There is now less death, so perhaps there is less money to be made in coffins, and more money to be made in expressing their talents through things of beauty for the living.

And even better, there was now a future – of their own making.

Irbil, Iraq
36°11′ N 44°1′ E

Columbus, Ohio
39°59′ N 82°59′ W

INTO OTHER LANDS

The volunteer flood down our gangway is flowing ever outward. In small but significant ways, we've begun to look for chances to partner in new areas of the world. In 2003, for instance, we joined a coalition of 173 other organisations and the United Nations in a massive operation to help Iraq after the overthrow of Saddam Hussein's government. Operation Iraqi Mercy was a collaborative effort with our partner German relief agency Humedica, that served thousands of people with practical assistance and promoted a message of reconciliation and friendship.

The team found four Kurdish children with conditions they couldn't cure there. So the team made a major commitment to provide them with the medical aid they needed. The two girls, aged nine and five, suffering from serious congenital heart defects, were flown with their fathers to Ohio. The other two, young brothers aged five and six, were victims of a land mine explosion. One lost his left arm and both boys suffered severe shrapnel wounds to the eyes.

In Ohio, a former Mercy Ships eye surgeon volunteer had enlisted his colleagues' expertise in an attempt to save them. Everyone waived fees, Mercy Ships paid travelling expenses, the Kurdish Humanitarian Rights Watch assisted in obtaining humanitarian parole visas, Airserv evacuated all four children and parents for free from Iraq to Jordan. Royal Jordanian Airlines offered a discount for the US portion of the flights.

And a whole merciful army of Ohioans pulled together to support the children's medical visit.

These and hundreds of other such Mercy Ships stories only happen because of the generous donors financially supporting the work and because of the almost one thousand volunteer crew and students from more than fifty countries who give time every year to offer their skills, talent, energy, and hearts to make it so.

Longitude/Latitude: From Everywhere

ADMIRALS OF MERCY

Who are these people who serve with Mercy Ships?

On a hospital ship, the medical work of healing the thousands who stream up our gangway is what gets most of the outward attention. In reality, that is only about 10 per cent of the actual work that makes a ship 'go'. The 90 per cent behind the scenes is what fuels the medical miracles on land and sea. Mercy Ships could not happen without every one of them.

Crew on the ships at any one time represent dozens of different nations – multicultural, multi-ethnic, multitalented.

English is the common language, and Catholic or Protestant Christianity in all its denominational variations – orthodox, main-line, evangelical, charismatic – is the predominant faith. There are also volunteers who have no religious persuasion, but want to help make the world a better place to live in.

Professional deckhands from both developed and developing nations keep the ships ship-shape. We have had a physical therapist from Portugal; an agricultural specialist from the United States; and a professional dancer from Trinidad, once recognised on the London dance scene, who was our media relations expert for most of our first twenty-five years.

A federal judge from the federal court in San Diego, California, has volunteered twice to be the ship's 'storesman'. He carries the 'stores' from where they are kept in cold and dry storage two decks below the galley, up the stairs and into the galley.

A blood relative of the Queen of England was part of our crew for five different visits to Africa. She was a part of the remarkable hospice team who visited those we could not help. The hospice team counselled the families on terminal care, not only bringing medical materials they could not afford, but also offering those individuals a greater dignity for the final months of their lives and to find peace in the midst of tragedy.

Her service along with others who continue to do hospice care has made one of the greatest statements Mercy Ships could make about the value of life – that the way we end our lives is important.

We have volunteers who have had their own lives transformed by the surgeries we specialise in – a nurse who had paediatric cornea transplant surgery now serves with us; a ship's officer who endured cleft lip and palate surgeries throughout his life. A woman from a long line of seafarers signed on as a third mate. A shipyard manager for an atomic submarine manufacturer became an executive officer. A teacher from England guides our multifaceted on-land operation.

We've had cooks from Norway, the United States, Ghana, and the Netherlands. And everyone onboard a ship knows that a crew's goodwill is directly proportional to the food they eat. If you have a good cook, you have a happy ship. If you don't have a good cook, you don't have a happy ship. So those who prepare the food, who wash the dishes, and who clean and do the service industry activities are a pivotal part of what make Mercy Ships International stay happily afloat.

They come from everywhere and every background, every ethnicity and nationality, even from other, stranded, ships. A Jamaican engineer was on a Russian ship in Mexican waters when the Russian ship went into bankruptcy. The crew onboard the ship were hungry. They couldn't go ashore because they were not Mexican citizens, so our crew, while we were in Lazaro Cardenas, began to help the crew stuck onboard. The Jamaican engineer asked if he could transfer to the Mercy Ship. We made arrangements with the agent ashore, and he joined us, and has been with us ever since.

Our very first captain was a former navy seal and a master mariner. Another of our captains was helping load equipment from his ship on to the *Caribbean Mercy*. 'This is something I would like to do with the rest of my life. I would love to raise my family onboard a ship,' he thought, after finding out more about us. And soon he and his family joined the crew.

The school onboard is one of the great strengths. The school on the *Anastasis*, for instance, has more than fifty students and at least seven full-time teachers, who meet during regular school-day hours. One of our educators was a teacher at one of England's most prestigious private schools.

From my perspective, the people who bring their families to serve onboard a Mercy Ship provide their children with an educational experience with an exposure to the globe unmatched by any university degree programme. The geography, the people, the languages, the cultures, the economic systems they see on a daily basis is unparalleled. I've seen its effect on my own children who have gone into their adult lives with an awareness of the world they could never have had through a conventional childhood on land.

I have always gathered people around me who were smarter than I am. In certain areas I think our organisation is close to genius. I am continually awed by the wonder-working gifts of the kind of person who becomes a ship's engineer. Watching one fix an average day's crises would convince anyone of that. But the same goes for anyone who chooses Mercy Ships as a career. Every one of our career volunteers seems able to do almost anything and actually looks for chances to do so – even our doctors.

Dr Gary Parker has served not only as the chief medical director of the *Anastasis* but also as its executive director. Yet that wasn't enough for this man. Case in point: While coming out of port in the Dominican Republic, not too long before we sailed to Africa in 1990, the *Anastasis* ran aground. This 11,701-ton ship was stuck, the propellers embedded in a coral reef behind us and in land in front of us. The propellers, by the way, even with the engines off, move with wave action. Since we were concerned that we were going to do even more serious damage to our propellers by forcing our way back into safe waters, someone had to go down and clear the path.

Who volunteered to don his scuba gear and clear the coral away from those massive but delicate propellers – which the waves are moving at will? Dr Gary Parker, whose hands should be insured for several million dollars, used those hands to get the ship sailing again. That tells you something about the kind of people who choose to spend a large part of their lives onboard a Mercy Ship.

As one Maritime Academy graduate has put it, 'Mercy Ships is more than the sea, and much more than just a job. It's my life.'

The sky is the limit; the sea is the road.

Mercy Ships staff and crew, those who have made Mercy Ships a career, are truly a rare group. From doctors to deckhands, everyone onboard pays his or her own way for the privilege of serving the poor. How is this done?

Crew raise their own support. An 'associate' crew member volunteers from two weeks to one year, either aboard ship or in one of our land-based offices. Crew range from eighteen-year-olds to retirees. Career crew members make a two-year commitment or longer. For those that make Mercy Ships a career, most of them raise their own financial support. For example, Dr Gary Parker, who came to help our efforts after the 1986 Mexico City earthquake for two weeks and has been with us ever since, asked his home church to sponsor him on that Mexico trip and they are still sponsoring him today.

I am convinced that this dynamic also fosters a real camaraderie, an *esprit de corps,* that goes beyond the people who actually get to be on the ship to those who support those who do. That's a powerful thing. And it's been a strong, quiet force in our success, and in the deep sense of fulfilment that is the hallmark of Mercy Ships.

Becoming a 'Shipmate' of Mercy Ships International is how thousands of people join Mercy Ships without leaving home. These are people who believe in what we are doing and pledge to help keep Mercy Ships International afloat, giving to us, as a charity, in the traditional way.

I've noticed a great dynamic at work in many of our volunteer crew and staff. Some were clearly on a pathway for success until they realised they wanted to do something more than become 'successful'. So, they took a turn onto the pathway of significance beyond success and found their way to us. The success/significance transition is a big one in the world today – the desire for legacy is a strong urge.

Actually, there is a theme of legacy throughout the whole Mercy Ships story, beginning with the Italian maritime leader who sold us the *Victoria,* which became the *Anastasis,* for a rock-bottom price. From the various captains, to the executive directors, to the able-bodied seamen, everyone involved with Mercy Ships is here for reasons having to do with leaving a meaningful legacy.

But surprisingly enough, the rewards come along the way. And sometimes they meet you at the door. Dr Keith Thomson, a consultant anaesthetist from the UK, experienced this in a fascinating way. During a visit to a maternity hospital in Sierra Leone as a volunteer, Dr Thomson found a nineteen-year-old woman in severe distress in the labour ward.

'What's wrong with this woman?' he asked the midwives.

The answer: 'She has been in labour for four days and she doesn't have the money for the Caesarian section that she needs.'

'Well, what will happen to her?' he asked.

The answer: 'She will probably die.'

'If I pay, will you do the surgery?' he asked.

The midwives asked the surgeon, who asked for a 20 per cent deposit of the total amount: the equivalent of one hundred dollars.

Dr Thomson paid it. The Caesarian section was performed, and a lovely little baby girl was born.

Five years later, Dr Thomson arrived at Conakry, Guinea's airport, to rejoin the *Anastasis.* As he left the airplane, he saw a couple with a child holding up a sign that said: 'Welcome, Uncle Keith. Thank you for saving my life and my mom's life. You are most welcome!'

Who are these people who have spent from two weeks to a lifetime to keep this dream of Mercy Ships afloat for a quarter of a century? Who have poured down our gangways to take fresh ideas, stubborn energy, and optimism into the lives of others – beyond all logic, beyond all statistics, beyond all reason and doubt?

Perhaps this one paragraph from a brochure for New Steps summarises the secret behind the Mercy Ships International success story better than I ever could:

> Committed individuals are needed to offer between three and twelve months to work. Positions available: prosthetists, technicians, physical and occupational therapists, social workers, project managers, skills trainers/micro enterprise developers, administrators. Qualities of compassion, patience, flexibility and perseverance are desirable.

The volunteers who fuel the Mercy Ships programmes on land and sea reflect that overflow of energy and heart and desire to put love into action. We exist today, and we face a bright future tomorrow because of them.

And we are, with small steps, with new steps, making a lasting difference, one person at a time.

SHIP'S LOG: APRIL 2005

Newcastle, England
55°2'N 1°42' W

As Wide As the Sea

Here I stand on the *Africa Mercy*, on a brisk day well into a new century, preparing for our 'shakedown' sail. The Blue Peter Flag has been lifted. I feel my heart catch in my throat.

I can see to the horizon everywhere I look, 360 degrees of deep blue.

And for a moment, I truly think I can see into the future – a ship called the *Asia Mercy*, a ship called the *Atlantic Mercy,* a Mercy Ship for every continent on this earth, each one with heart and hands to rival the ones who've steered us this far.

The rumble under my feet is a fine feeling – a feeling of energy, of hope, of life, and of power. And as I brace myself for the first full-out ride, I find myself thinking suddenly of four people, and I see their faces in the winds swirling all around me.

I see a girl named Edoh; I see my father; I see Mother Teresa; and I see my son J. P.

Edoh, the special Togolese girl whose story is our story in so many ways, has come back twice for follow-up surgeries since that day she was pitched over the fence into the hands of Mercy Ships crew member John Syrbe by the crushing but merciful crowd of fellow Togolese sufferers waiting for their own chance. The nine-year-old is now sixteen. Her father who sold everything to bring her the 500 kilometres to the Mercy Ship to save her life has now passed away. But despite her father's death putting her education in doubt, and with it her family's future, she has somehow not only stayed in school, but excelled. I can see her gazing around the ward where she spent so much time so many years ago, and hear her tell us that she wants to study nursing so she might join a Mercy Ship one day.

With only a look between us, Deyon and I and John pledged to support her education through high school and nursing school – if she truly wanted to go. And with bright eyes, she accepted. If Edoh does become a nurse, and ultimately serves on a Mercy Ship, I can think of nothing more thrilling or more fitting than seeing her in the medical wards of a ship exactly like this one.

And as the ship speeds up, I see my father and hear him saying: 'I am far more interested in the deeds of your life than any words you will ever say.'

I see Mother Teresa and hear her saying: 'Your son will help you on your journey to becoming the eyes, the ears, the mouth, and the hands for the poor.'

And I see J. P. and hear his silence that has spoken loudest of all.

My parents are gone now, and Mother Teresa is gone as well. My children are grown and have gone out into the world raising families and dreaming dreams of their own, while J. P. is still with us, on solid loving ground, still in need of constant daily care. He is now near the age I was when Mother Teresa spoke those words. And when I'm at home with J. P, as we go about our daily routine, offering our love by attending to his needs, I reflect on his life's impact on Mercy Ships' very existence, of his daily reminder to us of the value of the individual. It is a belief that has launched a growing fleet of ships and inspires so many to put their own words into action around the world. And I can't help but thank God for the privilege of it all – the privilege of the past, the privilege of this moment, and the privilege of the Mercy Ships yet to come.

Twenty-five years ago, all we had was a dream. But it was a powerful dream. More than ten thousand individuals from more than fifty nations have now walked the decks of a Mercy Ship, fuelling it on its merciful ways. And thousands upon thousands of individuals in the earth's neediest corners now await the Mercy Ship coming their way.

And so now we dream a new dream . . . a million people a year touched by hope and healing . . . a million dreams that have the power to come true.

The future is as wide as the sea.

In the words of Mother Teresa:

'Yesterday is gone.
Tomorrow has not yet come.
We have only today.
Let us begin.'

APPENDICES

APPENDIX I
ABOUT MERCY SHIPS INTERNATIONAL

A. AREN'T SHIPS EXPENSIVE TO OPERATE? (FINANCIAL LOGISTICS)

'Aren't ships expensive?'

We're often asked this question. And usually it is within the conext of a larger question: How do we do what we do so inexpensively? Mercy Ships International is known as one of the most efficient and effective charities afloat today, and we are often asked how we operate what seems to be an expensive concept so frugally.

In fact, operating ships can be incredibly inexpensive, if you do what we do. If you could take one of these big ships out of the water and stand it on its propellers, it would be a fifty-storey skyscraper. We operate the larger ships on approximately $3 million a year. If you divide that by the number of crew onboard (450), we operate these ships on less than $20 a day per person.

Because a Mercy Ship is in port 80–85 per cent of the time serving the poor, we only sail an average of fifty to fifty-five days per year. Our goal is to be in port ten months out of the year. Our steaming costs are a fraction of what it would be for a shipping company. In addition, our crew consists of volunteers who pay their own room and board to operate the ships. A completed audited annual report is available upon request, or may be viewed online at www.mercyships.org.

B. HOW DOES IT WORK? (PROGRAMMES AND STATISTICS)

Mercy Ships is a global charity, serving people of all faiths. We welcome volunteers who would like to give of their time, efforts, and expertise either on land or onboard ship to the work of bringing hope and healing to the world's poorest peoples. (See 'How can I get involved?' below.) Mercy Ships provides medical care, relief aid, and training for long-term sustainable change in developing nations. The following is a description of some of the services and pro-grammes that Mercy Ships currently provides:

Health Care Services

Highly skilled surgeons perform thousands of operations to remove tumours and cataracts, straighten crossed eyes, repair cleft lips and palates, correct fistulas, and provide a wide range of orthopaedic procedures. In most of the nations that Mercy Ships visits, these operations are often unavailable and/or unaffordable to the average person. Mercy Ships provides all services free of charge.

Mobile medical and dental teams establish field clinics in nearby communities to offer vaccination programmes, dental care, and minor operations. Mercy Ships supports the training of national doctors and nurses, and provides local people with education in hygiene, nutrition, and basic health care.

Community Development Services

In their commitment to facilitate long-term development in com-munities, Mercy Ships teams help construct hospitals, clinics, schools and vocational training facilities, homes, and churches. Offering training and advice, materials and hands-on assistance, Mercy Ships partners with local people and empowers communities to help themselves. Agricultural projects teach communities how to become more productive and efficient in growing food for them-selves and for the marketplace.

Animal husbandry projects, such as the 'Mercy Sheep' Project for Sierra Leone, help to replenish livestock levels and teach farmers basic animal care. Water and Sanitation teams test local water sources and train village representatives in how to break the water-borne disease cycle. They assist with individual and community latrine construction, and drill and rehabilitate wells to provide safe water for consumption and irrigation.

New Steps

Through the land-based New Steps team, dedicated health care pro-fessionals work with those who have lost limbs through land mines or atrocities of war. A primary focus of New Steps is working in various polio communities in Sierra Leone. New Steps focuses on serving the whole person by providing prosthetic limbs, physical and occupational therapy, counselling, family support, and vocational training.

Mercy Ships Nicaragua

Land-based Mercy Ships Nicaragua contributes to the long-term development of Nicaragua. They provide a training location dedi-cated to preparing volunteers from developing and developed nations with an emphasis on medical, relief, and community development.

C. WHAT HAS MERCY SHIPS ACCOMPLISHED?

Since 1978, Mercy Ships has performed more than 2 million services with a value of more than $250 million, and impacted more than 5.5 million people. While we work towards long-range solutions in these nations, our focus remains on helping individuals and communities. Some of the more notable statistics include:

- Performed more than 18,000 operations such as cleft lip and palate, cataract removal, straightening of crossed eyes, orthopaedic and facial reconstruction.

- Treated more than 300,000 people in village medical clinics.

- Performed 110,000 dental treatments.

- Taught over 5,500 local health care and professional workers, who have in turn trained multiple thousands in primary health care.

- Trained local medical professionals in modern health care techniques to carry on after the ship leaves.

- Delivered more than $21 million of medical equipment, hospital supplies, and medicines.

- Completed close to 350 construction and agriculture projects including schools, clinics, orphanages, and water wells.

- 850 career staff and crew from more than forty nations serve today.

- More than 1,600 short-term volunteers serve with Mercy Ships each year.

D. FAQs: FREQUENTLY ASKED QUESTIONS ABOUT MERCY SHIPS

What is Mercy Ships?

Mercy Ships is a global charity that serves people of all faiths. Mercy Ships provides health care services as well as community development services free of charge to those in desperate need. Highly skilled surgeons remove tumours and cataracts, straighten crossed eyes, repair cleft lips and palates, correct fistulas, and provide a wide range of orthopaedic procedures. Also, Mercy Ships teams help construct hospitals, clinics, schools, vocational training facilities, homes, and churches. Offering training and advice, materials and hands-on assistance, Mercy Ships partners with local people and other agencies. (See 'How does it work? Programmes and Statistics' above.)

Where are the ships and national offices?

Primarily the *Caribbean Mercy* operates in Central America and the Caribbean island nations, while the *Anastasis* and the *Africa Mercy* serve the poor in Africa. The next Mercy Ship is planned for Asia. To serve the growing fleet, national offices are located in North and Central America, Asia, Europe, Australia, and Africa. For an updated list of offices and contact information, or to find out where the ships are right now, visit us online: www.mercyships.org.

Where have the ships served?

The ships operate primarily in developing nations. From time to time, they also visit European or US ports to raise funds, procure supplies, and recruit volunteers. The nations where the ships have served outside of Europe and the USA include: Benin, Brazil, China, Cook Islands, Cuba, the Dominican Republic, El Salvador, Estonia, Faroe Islands, Fiji, The Gambia, Ghana, Grenada, Guatemala, Guinea, Guinea-Bissau, Guyana, Haiti, Honduras, Ivory Coast, Jamaica, Latvia, Liberia, Lithuania, Madagascar, Mexico, New Caledonia, New Guinea, Nicaragua, Papua New Guinea, the Philippines, Pitcairn Island, Poland, Samoa, Senegal, Sierra Leone, Solomon Islands, South Africa, South Korea, Togo, Tonga, Trinidad, and Vanuatu.

How much time do you spend in port or at sea?

An average of forty to sixty days per year are spent at sea. The rest of the time, the ships are docked in port, primarily in active service to the poor. For small amounts of time the ships conduct a public relations tour, where the emphasis is on recruiting volunteers and procuring supplies for upcoming field assignments.

What motivates your volunteers?

The majority of our crew would say that they are motivated to serve with Mercy Ships by an understanding of a loving God and understanding that the same loving God works through people to work for social justice and to bring a message of restoration.

Is Mercy Ships a Christian organisation and how does that affect its work?

Mercy Ships provides health care services and community development services to the poor in developing nations without prejudice or discrimination with regard to ethnicity, sex, age, or religion. Before we enter any nation, we sign a protocol with top government officials. In every nation where a Mercy Ship has served, including almost exclusively Muslim nations, we have been invited back and asked to return. There has never been any pressure or coercion on an individual to convert in order to receive services or help of any kind.

The foundational idea behind Mercy Ships was putting words into action as an expression of God's love, in the same spirit as Mother Teresa. People from diverse backgrounds and denominational affiliations staff Mercy Ships. Any person wishing to serve with Mercy Ships in a career capacity must agree with our core values. Mercy Ships welcomes volunteers, whatever their religious affiliation, who would like to be involved in the cause of meeting the needs of health and social justice for the world's poor, one person at a time. (See 'How can I get involved?' below.)

Who is Don Stephens and what is his background?

Don Stephens is the founder and president of Mercy Ships

International. He holds a bachelor's degree in religious studies from Bethany College, Santa Cruz, California, and has received the Two Hungers Award and the Religious Heritage Award. Don is the author of two books, *Trial by Trial* and *Mandate for Mercy*, and is a Paul Harris Fellow through Rotary. Married in 1966, Don and Deyon have four grown children and became grandparents in 2002. Conversant in German and French, Don lectures internationally and is the voice behind the *Mercy Minute*, a daily radio broadcast aired internationally on more 720 radio stations.

What is the relationship with Youth With A Mission?

Mercy Ships owes an immeasurable debt of gratitude to Youth With A Mission for its vital role in the birth and launching of Mercy Ships. In 2003, Mercy Ships and YWAM made a joint decision to be considered 'separate but equal' and no longer part of the same organisation. Mercy Ships and YWAM regularly collaborate and partner in a wide variety of projects throughout the world.

How is Mercy Ships funded?

The backbone of Mercy Ships is Shipmates. Through regular monthly donations, Shipmates makes the 'Acts of Mercy' possible. These 'Acts of Mercy', funded by Shipmates, help the blind see, the lame walk, and the poor receive news of the nature and character of a loving God.

In addition to Shipmates, Mercy Ships partners with a wide range of organisations that contribute finance, cargo, and services. Every dollar Mercy Ships receives is complemented by more than two dollars in contributed gifts-in-kind and services. The medical community donates pharmaceuticals, medical equipment, and supplies. Port fees are often waived. Most significantly, those serving on the ships pay for their room and board in monthly crew fees and raise their own finances to serve with Mercy Ships. For these reasons, the return on investment for Mercy Ships is nothing less than extraordinary.

How can I get involved?

Short-term volunteers can participate from two weeks to a full year with Mercy Ships, while others may choose to serve in a career capacity. People typically get involved either by volunteering to serve on a Mercy Ship or by making a decision to support the work with their funds. To do either of these, the next step involves contacting the Mercy Ships office in your country or region. Find out how to do that online at www.mercyships.org.

APPENDIX II
Mercy Ships' Vision, Accountability, Governance, Mission

Mercy Ships, a global charity, has operated a growing fleet of ships in developing nations since 1978. Following the example of Jesus, Mercy Ships brings hope and healing to the poor, mobilising people and resources worldwide.

Vision

Mercy Ships seeks to become the face of love in action, bringing hope and healing to the world's poor, with ships serving every continent of the world in the 21st century.

Values

The staff and crew of Mercy Ships International strive to live by several core values: 1. Love God; 2. Love and serve others; 3. Be people of integrity; 4. Be people of excellence in all that is said and done.

Accountability and Governance

Mercy Ships' core competencies are operating hospital ships and land-based sustainable development. Medicine and ships each require risk management. Independent, outside directors form the majority on the seventeen different legal boards around the world. The executive committee of the Mercy Ships International board has the primary responsibility for governance and accountability.

Outside directors bring significant expertise in medicine, shipping, business, finance, accounting, legal, and political arenas.

In 2003, the US Congress enacted new legislation for corporate directors, largely because of the Enron debacle. However, charitable organisations have also had their share of similar issues. The Sarbanes Oxley Act of 2003 has put in place new regulations to assure public trust.

However, prior to the Sarbanes Oxley Act, the chairman of the board of directors of Mercy Ships had already instituted the newly mandated regulations for business, and did so a year in advance. It is our view that transparency and accountability are high value currencies for the non-profit charitable sector, as well as corporate.

Under the leadership of our chairman, the following committees were established:

1. Nominating and Governance (overseeing diversity and board effectiveness)

2. Finance and Audit (overseeing independence, including an outside auditor)

3. Development (oversight and assistance on development and fund-raising)

4. Organisation (promoting independence on organisational matters)

5. Mission/Outreach (overseeing service delivery, training, and education)

Each Mercy Ships national office has its own governing board. The chairman of each national support board may be invited to serve with the outside directors of the International Board when certain national benchmarks are met. Each national support office signs an association agreement that aligns the policies and practices. In addition to the legal boards, there is an executive leadership team, consisting of the senior leadership positions within the organisation, for day-to-day management and operations. This executive leadership team carries out the direction set by the board and also gives recommendations and input to the board.

A charity as vast, multicultured, and multilayered as Mercy Ships International could only be performing in its existing global state through the direction of the remarkable people who are part of our ever-growing international board. What they all have in common are hearts full of charity, souls rich in service, and minds full of international medical, business, and personal experience offered gladly and wisely to the cause of serving the world's forgotten poor.

To view the latest list of board members of Mercy Ships, visit us online at www.mercyships.org in the 'About Us' section.

APPENDIX III
What World Leaders Say About Mercy Ships

We cannot thank you enough. Not only have you treated my people and taken care of them, but you have also taught them valuable lessons, the most important being love and respect and caring for each other irrespective of race and religion ... We Gambians are very grateful to you.

– A. J. Yahya Jammeh, **President, The Gambia**

Their work goes beyond healing and comforting the sick ... it provides a sense of hope that is badly needed in the places they work. I am delighted to give my support to Mercy Ships.

– Tony Blair, **Prime Minister, UK**

On behalf of the Honduran people, we would like to thank the staff and volunteers of Mercy Ships for the many touching moments of bringing care to our developing nation. The missions of Mercy Ships have been an example of hope, love and commitment. We have witnessed the purest form of compassion, giving without the slightest thought of compensation.

– Mary Flake de Flores
First Lady, the Republic of Honduras

It gives me great pleasure to express my support for this visionary enterprise of hospital ships bringing hope and healing to some of the world's most needy. – Jimmy Carter, **Former President, USA**

I wish ... to convey our deep gratitude for the love that you have for the population of Benin. To all of the ladies and gentlemen of the ship, I express my sincere congratulations for such an unflinching commitment on the side of the most vulnerable and poorest of third-world countries.

– MATHIEU KÉRÉKOU, **President, Benin**

Mercy Ships exemplifies for me a spirit of compassion for those in need. I personally am proud that in a world in which selfishness and greed are so often presented as prime motivators, Mercy Ships stands as a living antidote to self-interest.

– JOHN MAJOR, **Former Prime Minister, UK**

I feel very privileged that God gave me the opportunity to see that His work through men and women is ongoing daily. Today I have seen a ship and the men and women that take life, hope and dignity to the world. Thanks be to God.

– ALFONSO PORTILLO, **President, Guatemala**

For many years now, Mercy Ships has provided medical services for the poor throughout the world. You're reaching out to people in need – feeding the hungry, caring for the lonely, and giving urgent medical help to those who need it. I have every hope you will continue to reach more and more patients in the years beyond. I know you will continue your mission of bringing hope and healing to those who need it most. May God continue to bless you in your important work.

– GEORGE W. BUSH, **President, USA**

APPENDIX IV
SHIP SPECIFICATIONS

MV AFRICA MERCY
BUILT: HELSINGOR VAERFT, DENMARK, 1980
REGISTERED: MALTA
LENGTH: 152 METERS
BREADTH: 23.7 METERS
DAFT: 6 METERS
GROSS TONNAGE: 16,572
MAIN ENGINES: (4) B&W ALPHA DIESEL, 3120 KW EACH
AUXILIARY ENGINES: (2) B&W ALPHA DIESEL, 2800 KW EACH,
     (4) FRICHS, 750 KW EACH
CRUISING SPEED: 14 KNOTS
FUEL CAPACITY:1200 CU.M. APPROX.
FRESH WATER CAPACITY: 950 CU.M. APPROX.
CREW: 484
OPERATING THEATERS: 6

MV ANASTASIS
BUILT: TRIESTE, ITALY 1953
REGISTERED: MALTA
LENGTH: 159 METERS
BREADTH: 20.7 METERS
DAFT: 7.2 METERS
GROSS TONNAGE: 11,701
MAIN ENGINES: (2). FIAT 7510, 10 CYL., 8050 BHP EACH
AUXILIARY ENGINES: (2) WARTSILA 4R22/28, 540 KW EACH,
     (2) DAIHATSU DL20, 600 KW EACH
CRUISING SPEED: 14 KNOTS
FUEL CAPACITY: 1490 CU.M.
FRESH WATER CAPACITY:1050 CU.M.
CREW: 410
OPERATING THEATERS: 4

MV CARIBBEAN MERCY
BUILT: AALBORG, DENMARK, 1952
REGISTERED: PANAMA
LENGTH: 79.8 METERS
BREADTH: 12.2 METERS
DAFT: 4.5 METERS
GROSS TONNAGE: 2,152
MAIN ENGINE: (1) MAK DIESEL, 3670 BHP
AUXILIARY ENGINES: (2) CATERPILLAR, 320 KW EACH
CRUISING SPEED: 14 KNOTS
FUEL CAPACITY:154 CU.M.
FRESH WATER CAPACITY:120 CU.M.
CREW: 150
OPERATING THEATERS: 2

Africa Mercy

Deck 5   Deck 4   Deck 3

Africa Mercy

Deck 8   **Deck 7**   **Deck 6**

Anastasis

A Deck   B Deck   C Deck

Anastasis

Bridge Deck   **Lido Deck**   **Promenade Deck**   **Upper Deck**

Funnel Deck

Caribbean Mercy

A Deck B Deck C Deck

Funnel Deck

Caribbean Mercy
Boat Deck   Promenade Deck

ABOUT THE AUTHOR

DON STEPHENS is the founder and President of Mercy Ships. Winner of numerous awards, Don lectures internationally and is the voice behind the 'Mercy Minute', a daily radio broadcast aired around the globe.

Other books published by Hodder & Stoughton:

God's Smuggler

Brother Andrew

Since its publication in the late sixties, more than ten million people have read *God's Smuggler*. The adventure-packed, inspirational true story tells of Brother Andrew's journey from humble beginnings to a worldwide mission to bring Bibles to Christians cut off from the Church.

ISBN 0 340 86114 2

Light Force

Brother Andrew with Al Janssen

When the phenomenal success of *God's Smuggler* made it too dangerous for his contacts in the underground church, Brother Andrew decided he could not return to Eastern Europe. For the last thirty-five years he has been serving the Christian Church in the Middle East as well as witnessing to Jews and Muslims.

Light Force brings Brother Andrew's story right up to date. It is every bit as exciting as *God's Smuggler*, as Andrew continues to put his life on the line.

ISBN 0 340 86272 6

Corrie ten Boom

In My Father's House:
The Years before The Hiding Place

Concentrating upon her family and their life in Holland before the
war, this inspiring and revealing book describes in moving detail
living above the family watch shop in Harlem and her memories of
the family together before their lives changed for ever with the
advent of war and persecution. Corrie believed that her early
life gave her the strength to survive the war, brutal hardship
and persecution, and to begin her worldwide ministry.

ISBN 0 340 86375 7

The Hiding Place

Still a bestseller more than thirty years after first publication,
The Hiding Place is Corrie ten Boom's memoir of how her family
protected Jews during the Nazi occupation of Holland, and the
horrors of the Holocaust. Despite the danger and threat
of discovery and their arrest, they courageously offered
shelter to persecuted Jews.

ISBN 0 340 86353 6

Tramp for the Lord:
The Years after The Hiding Place

Tramp for the Lord tells of Corrie's experiences after the Second
World War. She began to minister worldwide and travel widely,
visiting those she felt were suffering and who were in need of
leading to the Lord in places as diverse as Africa and Germany.
An impressive and inspiring book telling Corrie's story in the
years after the events of the bestselling *Hiding Place*.

ISBN 0 340 86376 5

Fatwa

Jacky Trevane

The amazing story of a woman who risked her life to get herself
and her two little girls out of Cairo and away from an abusive
husband. Now back in the UK, Jacky is still living in the shadow
of a Fatwa, a Muslim death threat. She has to protect herself
and her daughters constantly. This memoir will ensure that
her story is never forgotten . . .

ISBN 0 340 86242 4

Hidden Sorrow, Lasting Joy

Anneke Companjen

Anneke Companjen, wife of the President of Open Doors
International, tells the true stories of twenty contemporary
Christian women from all around the world. Some suffer direct
persecution for what they believe. Others are the wives, mothers
and daughters of the men who are imprisoned, tortured
and murdered. Every story is unique, challenging,
shocking and inspiring.

ISBN 0 340 75675 6

Prisoners of Hope

Dayna Curry and Heather Mercer

Dayna Curry and Heather Mercer tell the story of their work in Afghanistan, their love for the people they served, their arrest, trial, imprisonment by the Taliban, and their rescue in the midst of war by US Special Forces. The book discusses how two middle-class American women decided to leave the comforts of home in exchange for the opportunity to serve the disadvantaged, and how their faith motivated and sustained them through the events that followed.

ISBN 0 340 86121 5

Street Children of Brazil

Sarah de Carvalho

This is the remarkable true story of a life transformed. Sarah de Carvalho left her successful career in film and TV, and joined a missionary organisation in Brazil. There she met children living on the streets, struggling to survive.

This is a story of immense faith, suffering and love. The children whose stories are revealed in this exceptional book will change the heart of every reader.

ISBN 0 340 64164 9